DR. McDOUGALL'S

Digestive Tune-Up

John A. McDougall, MD

ILLUSTRATIONS BY HOWARD BARTNER

HEALTHY LIVING PUBLICATIONS

Summertown, Tennessee

Library of Congress Cataloging-in-Publication Data

McDougall, John A.
  Dr. McDougall's digestive tune-up / John A. McDougall ; illustrations by
Howard Bartner.
     p. cm.
  Includes bibliographical references and index.
  ISBN-13: 978-1-57067-184-5
  ISBN-10: 1-57067-184-2
  1. Digestive organs--Diseases--Diet therapy--Popular works. 2. Digestive
organs--Diseases--Nutritional aspects--Popular works. 3. Nutrition--Popular
works. 4. Vegetarianism--Popular works. I. Title.
   RC806.M23 2006   616.3'0654--dc22

15 14 13 12 11 10 09 08   2 3 4 5 6 7 8 9 10

© 2006, 2008 John A. McDougall, MD

Illustrations: *Howard Bartner*
Cover and interior photos: *Ed Aiona*
Design: *Aerocraft Charter Art Service*

Printed in Canada.

Healthy Living Publications
a division of Book Publishing Company
P.O. Box 99
Summertown, TN 38483
888-260-8458

ISBN 10: 1-57067-184-2
ISBN 13: 978-1-57067-184-5

Book Publishing Co. is a member of Green Press Initiative. We chose to print this title
on paper with postconsumer recycled content, processed without chlorine, which
prevented the following waste of natural resources:

9 tons of wood
2,919 pounds of solid waste
22,120 gallons of water
5,329 pounds of greenhouse gases
42 million BTU of energy

For more information, visit <www.greenpressinitiative.org>. Savings calculations thanks to the
Environmental Defense Paper Calculator, <www.papercalculator.org>.

Contents

Before You Begin   v
AN IMPORTANT NOTE FROM DR. MCDOUGALL

Acknowledgments   *vii*

Introduction   *ix*

CHAPTER 1 Sickness, Stroke,
and a Brand New Start   1

CHAPTER 2 Meet the Patients   5
THE BORTONS TELL ALL

CHAPTER 3 Bad Breath   11
MUCH MORE THAN MEETS THE NOSE

CHAPTER 4 My Stomach's on Fire
and I Can't Put It Out   23

CHAPTER 5 What's Eating You?   37
SAYING SO LONG TO ULCERS

CHAPTER 6 Here's to a Happy Gallbladder   49

CHAPTER 7 The Liver to the Rescue   61

CHAPTER 8 In Search of the Perfect
Bowel Movement   69

CHAPTER 9   Bowel Sickness
and the Fiber Factor   91

CHAPTER 10   Chained to the Bathroom
with Colitis   93

CHAPTER 11   Colon Polyps and Cancer   107
THE GUT SAYS, "ENOUGH!"

CHAPTER 12   Beneficial Bowel Bacteria   117
OUR NEGLECTED FRIENDS

CHAPTER 13   Flatulence   127
EXPLORING THE F-WORD

CHAPTER 14   Evolution, Anatomy,
and Proper Human Nutrition   135

CHAPTER 15   Shopping, Cooking,
and Comfort Foods Galore   143

Notes   *159*

Reference   *189*

Index   *205*

Before You Begin

This instructional material offers you a significant opportunity to regain your health and enhance your personal appearance. However, diet is powerful medicine. Do not change your diet or start an intense exercise program if you are seriously ill or on medication, unless you are under the care of a physician knowledgeable in nutrition and its effects on health. Do not change medications without professional advice. When appropriate, share this message with your doctor. If abnormal bowel movements persist after a change to a plant-based diet, especially if there is accompanying pain or bleeding, a doctor's examination is indicated.

The McDougall Diet is a pure-vegetarian diet based around starchy vegetables, with the addition of fresh or frozen fruits and other vegetables. If you follow this diet strictly for more than three years, or if you are pregnant or nursing, you should take a minimum of five micrograms (mcg) of supplemental vitamin B_{12} each day.

Even though this instructional material is quite complete for changing your life, there is much more information to be found on the McDougall Web site at www.drmcdougall.com and in the McDougall books. Between the Web site and books you will find over 2,200 recipes to choose from. One of the most helpful and cost-effective experiences you can have is to view a McDougall DVD seminar. However, those of you desiring serious change in your health and medical care should consider becoming involved in one of the many programs at the McDougall Health Center. During the ten-day live-in McDougall Program you will become a patient of Dr. McDougall's. In this controlled and comfortable environment, you will rapidly progress to become medication-free, trim, active, healthy, and feeling better than you ever thought possible.

Contact Us

E-mail: office@drmcdougall.com

Web site: www.drmcdougall.com

The McDougall Health Center
PO Box 14039
Santa Rosa, CA 95402

Telephone: (800) 941-7111 or (707) 538-8609
FAX: (707) 538-0712

Acknowledgments

The bowels lie deep inside the body—shrouded by a cloak of mystery, trimmed with a sash of shame. On the pages that follow, I hope to remove the cloak and strip away the shame. I will speak frankly about subject matters that some may find delicate, even offensive. Because of my commitment to tell this story in a candid manner, three writers refused to work with me. Finding the right publisher was no small task either, taking three years to discover a company that shared my vision for a straightforward, practical discussion aimed at helping people live healthier, fuller lives. My goal is not to offend but to empower.

Those brave people joining me in this journey into the depths of the gut deserve some special recognition. First and foremost, writer Lisa Espinoza spent hundreds of hours translating my dry technical language into a warm and entertaining story. She brought unmatched talent and dedication to this project.

Medical illustrator Howard Bartner provided the humorous drawings of Larry and Louise used throughout the book. Darryl Lujo, a talented medical illustrator and friend of Howard Bartner, provided digital expertise to enhance the images.

My gratitude goes to Bob and Cynthia Holzapfel, publisher and managing editor at Book Publishing Company, for their willingness to make the extra stretch and publish a book on this untouchable subject. Jo Stepaniak was responsible for copyediting. John Wincek deserves credit for the cover and interior design of the book.

Thanks to the efforts of these and other talented people, read-ers will now have the opportunity to make simple dietary choices and well-informed medical decisions that will bring health to their intestinal tract, the portal to the rest of the body.

Introduction

I f you've picked up this book, chances are you suffer from the same nagging symptoms as most Americans—bloating, indigestion, chronic abdominal pain after eating, frequent diarrhea, or the opposite, constant constipation. Maybe you've even been diagnosed with one of the plethora of digestive disorders plaguing our society—gallbladder disease, irritable bowel syndrome (IBS), diverticulosis, Crohn's disease, gastroesophageal reflux disease (GERD), or ulcerative colitis, just to name a few. Or perhaps you're just curious. Good. Prevention is always the preferred option. If you're in the unfortunate bellyaching group, take heart—you're about to discover a plan for rescuing your ailing body. No doubt you've heard the old antacid pitch, "How do you spell relief?" You're about to learn a new way to spell relief, and it doesn't come in a pill.

I'm going to make a statement that may surprise you. You may even doubt its validity at first. Although it makes perfect sense, it has been concealed by

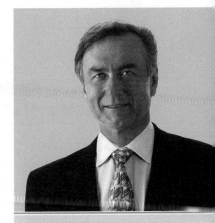

I'm the luckiest doctor in the world because my patients regain their lost health and appearance by following the simple, cost-free, side-effect-free dietary and lifestyle advice I prescribe.

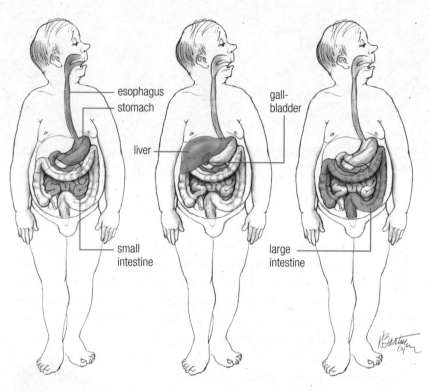

UPPER INTESTINAL TRACT   LOWER INTESTINAL TRACT

Our journey through the intestinal tract will be in three stages: first the upper intestinal tract, then the liver and gallbladder, and finally the lower intestine.

controversy originating from those who stand to lose the most if you stumble upon the truth. And here is the truth—the food you put into your body is the *single* most powerful factor that determines your health and well-being. How can I make this bold claim? The answer will soon be clear.

On the pages that follow, you will read my story—how I was transformed from a chronically ill young man to a person who could be considered the picture of health. At fifty-nine years of age (I was born in 1947), I continue to reap the benefits of fueling my body with the right foods. How many grandpas do you know who regularly windsurf in the deep blue ocean or strap their grandson into a backpack to carry him on a mountainous hiking adventure? Because of proper diet, this is the kind of health I enjoy today.

You'll also meet two of my patients, Larry and Louise Borton, who likewise found their way back to health by following the same plan that revolutionized my life. Their story is retold again and again in the hundreds of patients I've seen restored to good health and vitality during my thirty years of medical practice. Through dietary change, these individuals have experienced improvement in all aspects of their health, including lower blood pressure and cholesterol levels, relief from headaches and arthritis pain, and even, in many cases, complete healing of diseases as serious as type 2 diabetes, obesity, rheumatoid arthritis, and heart disease (actually reversing atherosclerosis) *without* medication. In this book we will focus our discussion on issues related to the digestive system—how it works, what can go wrong, and most importantly, what we can do to make you well again.

I am confident that when you choose to follow the dietary principles and lifestyle changes I am about to share with you, you will soon be saying good-bye to the belly and bowel problems that have been plaguing you. And I am confident that you will experience dramatic improvement in your overall health—looking and feeling better than ever.

CHAPTER 1

Sickness, Stroke, and a Brand New Start

Images of a little brown-haired boy curled into a fetal position on the couch punctuate the otherwise pleasant memories of my childhood. Excruciating stomachaches and severe constipation intruded upon my daily life, making carefree boyhood activity virtually impossible. As a teenager, I came to expect acid indigestion and reflux as the last course of my usual lunch of ring bologna on white bread washed down with a half-gallon of whole milk. Because daily stomach distress was all I'd ever known, I thought the constant pain from the top to the bottom of my intestines was normal.

As an eighteen-year-old freshman in college, I suffered a major stroke, a condition that strikes about a thousand teenagers annually in the United States. The stroke caused paralysis of the entire left side of my body. Two weeks after this damage to my brain, I was able to move my left thumb one-quarter inch—an accomplishment that in my estimation meant it was time to discharge myself from Grace Hospital in Detroit, Michigan. After several months, I recovered about 60 percent of my strength and coordination. Still today I walk with a noticeable limp.

At twenty-two years of age, during my medical school training, my body, belly, and butt ached like someone two or three times my age. To add insult to injury, when I reached my all-time highest weight of two hundred twenty-eight pounds at six feet tall, I was so heavy that even my own mother called me fat.

A few years later, as a twenty-five-year-old intern at Queens Medical Center in Honolulu, Hawaii, the stomach pains that had been my lifelong companion became so intense that they often forced me to curl up with cramps after my dinner. Finally, at my wife Mary's insistence, I consulted a doctor. Unfortunately, I was doing my surgery rotation that month, so the opinion I sought was that of a surgeon. You can guess where I spent that afternoon—undergoing exploratory abdominal surgery for what my doctors thought was appendicitis. Peering into my wide-open abdominal cavity, the doctors found a perfectly healthy appendix, but chose to remove it anyway for good measure. No one before or after my surgery ever inquired about the three chili dogs I ate before bedtime each evening.

If my second quarter of life was to be any reflection of my first, I would almost certainly be plagued with hemorrhoids, diverticulitis, hiatus hernia, stomach ulcers, and maybe a heart attack or another stroke. And, *if* I survived, it was anybody's guess as to what the golden years would bring—maybe bypass surgery and colon cancer. Fortunately, this dismal future was only a product of my speculation. I rewrote the inevitable ending to my story when, as a sick young man of twenty-seven, I chose to make a drastic lifestyle change. Now, at almost sixty years of age, I enjoy far better health than I did even as a teenager.

The turning point in my life came soon after finishing my internship at Queen's Medical Center. My first job was as a family practitioner caring for approximately five thousand workers at the Hamakua Sugar Plantation on the Big Island of Hawaii. Being one of only four doctors practicing in the countryside, my responsibilities were unusually broad. I attended to life from beginning to end—delivering babies, repairing injuries, refilling monthly prescriptions, providing hospital care, and pronouncing people dead. As a result, I became a very experienced doctor, and most of my patients fared well. However, these remarkable people gave back to me a gift far greater than I could have hoped to give them—they taught me the *truth* about proper human nutrition.

My patient population consisted mostly of first, second, third, and fourth-generation Japanese, Chinese, Koreans, and Filipinos. In this multigenerational mix of patients I began to observe distinct patterns. The first generation were always trim, usually active into their nineties, and never suffered from constipation, hemorrhoids, ulcers, diabetes, heart disease, or cancers of the breast, prostate, or colon. However, their children and grandchildren began to exhibit these types of Western illnesses that were almost nonexistent in their healthy parents and grandparents. What was the difference?

There was only one fundamental factor that could account for the increasing gap between the excellent health of the first generation and the progressively deteriorating health of the second, third, and fourth generations. That factor was diet. My first generation patients had remained faithful to their native starch-based diet (mainly rice) with the addition of fruits and vegetables. Their offspring born in Hawaii, however, began to incorporate more rich Western foods into their diets while decreasing their consumption of starches (rice), fruits, and vegetables. They gained weight and became sicker. This observation served as a catalyst for profound changes in both my personal and my professional life.

As I learned more about nutrition and began incorporating this age-old wisdom into my own eating habits, it

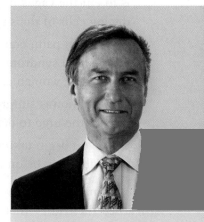

I've earned the right to talk to you about the harms caused to a person's health by eating a rich diet—I almost died as a result of this. Now at nearly sixty, I am healthier and more active than I was in my mid-twenties.

became clear to me that diet was indeed the foundation for good health. I quickly began feeling better. The digestive problems that had tormented me since childhood became a thing of the past.

As I reflected upon my lifelong quest for relief from within the medical community, I wondered why no one had ever asked me the simple question, "John, what do you *eat* every day?" And why was it that I *never* heard anything about this food/health connection in all my years of medical training? How could something as fundamental and obvious as what went into my mouth at least three times a day be overlooked as a source of my incessant indigestion, cramps, and constipation? Well, it was. In fact, the notion that food has a direct impact on health is adamantly denied in the following samples of what I was taught in medical school about digestive health:

- Stomach ulcers are not caused by diet but rather by the emotional stresses of life, and the solution to these painful craters is to cut the vagus nerve connecting the brain to the acid-producing cells of the stomach.
- Abdominal pain, cramps, and diarrhea (commonly called irritable bowel syndrome) are symptoms of neurosis common to middle-age women and are best treated by tranquilizers.
- Constipation is simply a learned behavior caused by failure to answer the urge to defecate.
- Once you begin taking medications for digestive problems, you will likely be on them for the rest of your life.

Fortunately, through intense research and firsthand experience, I learned the truth—that each of these "sound" medical assertions was dangerously erroneous. As we begin our journey through the digestive system, you too will recognize the absurdity of these claims. You will understand how your digestive system functions and how it reacts to the foods you eat. You will become a well-informed consumer, equipped and motivated to make healthful dietary choices rather than taking at face value the medical claims that can keep you curled up on the couch or standing in line at the drugstore to buy potions and pills.

Given this newfound knowledge about nutrition and health from my sugar plantation experience, it was impossible for me to practice medicine the way I'd been taught. Despite scathing criticism and obvious efforts by colleagues to divert my enthusiasm, my resolve was steadfast. I would care for patients, but I would be a different kind of doctor—one who would empower my patients with the knowledge and ability to be truly well. I would do all that I could do to keep another little brown-haired boy from lying curled up on the couch in pain when he should be outside playing.

CHAPTER 2

Meet the Patients

THE BORTONS TELL ALL

Discussion of the bowels and their contents is far down on the list of fun things to chat about (except in junior high circles, of course). Furthermore, when the need for such a discussion arises, people are tentative and unsure how to express themselves for fear of being deemed inappropriate. For the sake of comfort and propriety, the true story about our bowels might best be left untold. However, for the sake of the millions suffering with debilitating diseases of the intestine, the story *must* be told. To bring this sensitive subject to light, I have enlisted the help of two of my patients.

Larry and Louise Borton, both in midlife, came to my office a little over two years ago with a mile-long list of ailments reaching from one end of the digestive tract to the other. To say these two are not bashful is an understatement. With no more prodding than a casual *So what brings you here today?* Larry and Louise took turns rattling off every intimate detail about their health and their bodies. They had seen many other doctors and reported taking a cabinet full of prescription and nonprescription drugs in pursuit of relief from their symptoms. Despite trying every fad diet imaginable, both remained overweight and in poor health.

Louise was born and raised in Detroit, Michigan. Her mother and father are still living and in fairly good health. Louise teaches seventh grade and told me when we first met that she loved the students but found the politics of teaching to be very stressful.

5

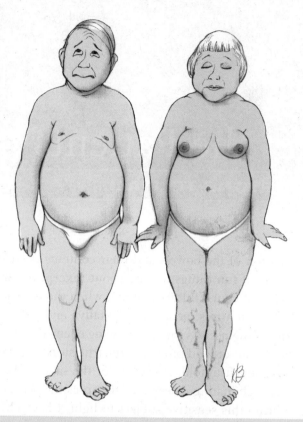

Larry Borton—age: 54, weight: 210 pounds, height: 5 feet, 7 inches
Louise Borton—age: 50, weight: 170 pounds, height: 5 feet, 5 inches

Larry was raised in San Francisco. After graduating from the University of California, Berkeley, he joined a software company in Silicon Valley. Life has been more difficult since the dot-com fall of 2000, and Larry said he was thankful to still be employed. The Bortons have been married twenty-seven years and make their home in San Jose, California. Their two children are grown and live nearby, giving Larry and Louise ample opportunity to spoil their three grandchildren.

When Larry and Louise first came to me for a consultation two years ago, their chief concerns were about my qualifications. "Why should we listen to you?" Larry asked. Louise added, "What makes you different from all the other diet experts who say theirs is the only right way to eat?" "Yeah," interrupted Larry, "we've tried everything from Atkins to Fit for Life."

Without thinking, I robotically rattled off my credentials, "I am a medical doctor, a board certified internist." Both Larry and Louise waited to hear more. Their experiences had taught them that traditionally trained doctors have little to offer when it comes to sound nutritional advice. Research bears this out—a 1990 published study suggests that only about one-quarter of medical schools require training in the medical nutrition sciences, and of those medical schools that offer nutrition electives, many achieve low enrollments.

I decided to share with the Bortons my own personal journey, how I was restored to health through dietary change, and how I'd seen the same successful story played out over and over in patients just as sick as and even sicker than they were.

A New Way of Thinking about Food

Larry and Louise appreciated me sharing my story. But they weren't quite convinced that diet alone could make that kind of dramatic difference in their health.

"Look around the world," I began, "and you will notice that the trimmest, healthiest, most youthful people live on plant-based, high-carbohydrate diets." The Bortons looked skeptical. "To be more specific," I continued, "Asians follow diets based on rice with vegetables, and the trim people from Peru eat mostly potatoes. People living in rural Mexico live primarily on corn and beans while those in Africa thrive on millet and beans. In New Guinea, sweet potatoes are the mainstay, and in the Middle East, chickpeas and rice are the dietary staples."

Louise countered, "These people work hard in the fields all day long, so how do you know the benefits are from their diet and not all that hard work and exercise?"

Good point. "Louise, many of these people living in underdeveloped countries have sedentary jobs. They work as school

Through your intestines you directly contact the outside world. You may have thought of your bowels as being inside your body. In reality, they are outside. Picture a tire tube. The inner surfaces facing the center are still "outside." To get inside the tube you would have to puncture the rubber. Now stretch that tube out thirty feet, the length of your intestine, and you can see that the intestine really is an outside surface that contacts the environment (food) directly. This intimate connection will help you understand why the foods you choose have such an immediate effect on the intestines.

teachers, shopkeepers, religious leaders, and accountants, and they are all trim and free of the diseases so common in America."

"Maybe it's genetic," offered Larry.

"Well, if it were genetic, then even when these people migrate to a Western nation, like the United States or the countries of Europe, they would retain their history of good health. That's just not the case. When people raised on a plant-based, high-carbohydrate diet begin consuming less carbohydrate and more fat and protein, like their Western counterparts, they gain weight and become sicker." The Bortons sat in rapt attention.

"Similar changes in health are seen within nations like Japan, as the people become wealthy from industrialization and begin to eat more rich American foods. Along with weight gain, their cholesterol levels rise, and then heart disease, diabetes, and arthritis become an expected part of everyday life—just like in the United States."

Larry and Louise's show-me-what-you've-got attitude gave way to cautious hopefulness.

"That makes sense, Dr. McDougall," said Larry. "I'm still not going to get my hopes up too much, but if you can do something about the constant bloating, the constipation one day and diarrhea the next, I'm in."

Louise nodded enthusiastically in agreement. "If you can help us throw away the cabinet full of pills and potions that do nothing but take up space, we'll have you over for prime rib and cheesecake to celebrate."

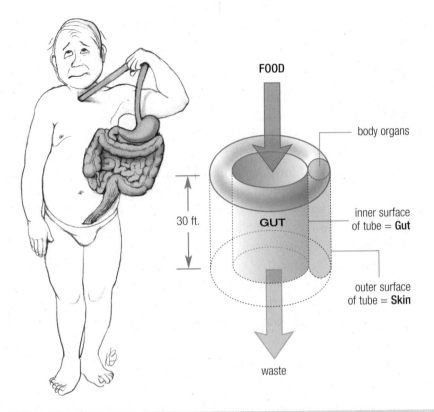

FOOD

body organs

inner surface
of tube = **Gut**

30 ft.

GUT

outer surface
of tube = **Skin**

waste

This comparison with a tire tube helps explain how our intestines have direct contact with the outside world. Think of your guts as being outside of your body, like the inner surface of a tire tube.

The Bortons had a lot to learn, but they were ready to take the first step. "Larry and Louise, I accept your invitation, but let's not plan the menu just yet."

I was thrilled to know the Bortons were soon going to experience better health than ever before. There was a reason why they felt poorly and were falling apart far too young. Fortunately, the human body can heal itself in miraculous ways if given the chance. This was the Bortons' chance.

The best place to begin a journey for healing is right where the primary symptoms lie—in the digestive system. After all, the bowels are the portal to the rest of the body through which every drop of water, calorie of energy, and body-building nutrient enters—and, let's not forget to mention, an assortment of toxins that can damage the brain, bones, liver, and heart.

My dealings with the Bortons and their digestive problems will act as a framework for our dialogue. They are open and honest, ask good questions, and unfortunately have suffered with most of the intestinal illnesses that we will be talking about. As any doctor in the general practice of medicine will tell you, Larry and Louise's health issues are not uncommon, and you will likely recognize yourself or someone you know within their story. As with the Bortons, this is your chance to regain your health and to feel better than you ever thought possible. We'll start at the top—the mouth—and work our way through the digestive system to the obvious end. Then I will equip you, just as I did the Bortons, with the practical information you need to begin today cooking and enjoying the nutritious foods that will serve as the foundation for a vital, healthy life.

CHAPTER 3

Bad Breath

MUCH MORE THAN MEETS THE NOSE

During their first visit, Larry confided that he had received more than a few painful comments from friends about his breath. Louise explained, "I've never noticed it myself, but the other day our little grandson asked, 'Papa, why is there a yucky smell in your mouth?'"

Apparently, the Bortons aren't the only ones concerned about halitosis (the kinder, gentler term for bad breath). From gum to mints, toothpaste to mouthwash and even entire oral hygiene systems, the abundance of products promising clean, fresh breath bears witness to the fact that we are indeed a nation highly concerned about the odors emanating from our mouths. In fact, between 50 and 60 percent of people in Western countries reportedly suffer from chronic bad breath—the rest sadly have not one honest friend who will tell them the truth.

But is bad breath really inevitable? As its more formal moniker suggests, halitosis (*hali* meaning breath *tosis* meaning an abnormal or diseased condition) is not necessarily a normal state. As Larry and Louise were soon to find out, by making adjustments in just two areas—oral hygiene practices and eating habits—you can virtually eliminate malodor of the mouth and maintain a consistently pleasant breath quality. This important change signals an even greater fundamental reality—you have become a healthier individual.

The Significance of Smells

We willingly fork over $45 for a three-ounce bottle of scented liquid to be dabbed here and there and emptied in three months because we want to smell good. We load our grocery carts with fresh-scented deodorants, fruity-smelling shower gels, and minty-fresh toothpastes because we know that how we smell sends a lasting message about ourselves. Multibillion-dollar fragrance industries know what we know—smell matters.

Your personal body scents leave an impression with everyone you meet about who you are. They affect your desirability as a friend and as a mate. This isn't just a sentiment shared by only a shallow few. It's hardwired into our brains. To help Larry and Louise understand what I meant by this, I asked them to recall one of their first encounters together.

"You mean like when I took Louise to the livestock show at the county fair?" Larry inquired.

"Well, yes, or perhaps you can recall a time that was a bit more . . ."

Louise chimed in, "*Romantic* is what he's trying to say, Larry. Dr. McDougall, I remember once when Larry took me on a date to a nice Italian restaurant. He showed up with carnations, looking handsome as could be in his khakis and button-up shirt, hair all combed back like James Dean—yes, he did have hair back then."

"Do you remember what he smelled like, Louise?"

"Are you kidding—to this day I can't resist giving him a little smooch when he dabs on his Old Spice cologne. It always takes me back to that special night."

I probed further, "And what about you, Larry—what do you remember about Louise on that date?"

"I'm not too good with details, but I do remember she looked drop-dead gorgeous. And when I leaned over to kiss her on the cheek, I couldn't believe how good her hair smelled. I wanted to touch it, but I was a gentleman."

"Ever smell anything similar since that night, Larry?"

"Now that you mention it, yeah. It's really weird though. I don't know if he uses the same shampoo or what, but every time this one waiter at Denny's bends over to give me my coffee I get flashbacks of Louise and the flowers and wishing I could touch her hair. Am I losing it?"

"Not at all," I answered. "This is what I meant by our brains being hardwired for smells." I went on to explain to the Bortons how this works.

When aromas enter through our nostrils, they stimulate over ten million sensory nerves located on the olfactory lobes of the brain. These lobes, or branches, of the brain carry messages via nerve fibers directly to an area of the brain called the *limbic system*, dedicated to processing our most intimate emotions including love, sexual desire, and anger.

Various scents produce subtle but profound arousals that can change your entire life. For example, the power of aromas given off by a woman's body at the time of her ovulation is scientifically documented to heighten her attractiveness to a man, thereby taking advantage of her fertility and leading to a greater chance of her mating successfully. Louise insisted that a simple *Good morning!* was all Larry needed to produce a greater chance of mating.

This "scentual" communication goes both ways. Women in the fertile phase of their cycle prefer the body odor of dominant men. This preference varies with relationship status, being much stronger in fertile women in stable relationships than in fertile single women. According to the theory, single women are most interested in stable relationships with men who will make great fathers. Once this security is established, an innate urge emerges to search for the best genes found in the most dominant men. Even without our realizing it, our natural bodily smells act as powerful avenues of communication.

If You Eat It, You Ooze It

Once I had established the groundwork for how smells influence us, the Bortons and I moved on to how we can influence our smells. Food is a major determining factor in how we smell to others. It's easy to pinpoint the guy in the office who just lunched on garlic chicken or a burger with onions (unless, of course, you have likewise indulged). Stories are often told of how

LIMBIC SYSTEM = EMOTION

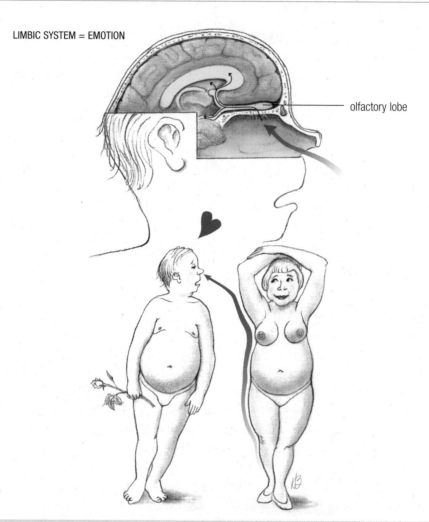

olfactory lobe

Messages of sexual desire, love, anger, and much more are communicated by our body odors. Carry on a friendlier exchange with those close to you by eating pleasant-smelling foods.

Eskimos smell similar to the fish they consume in their daily diet. During the Vietnam War, Vietnamese soldiers reported they could readily identify and target American soldiers traveling upwind by their dissimilar smell, a direct result of regular meat and dairy product consumption.

I first noticed this connection between foods and body odor during my early days of practice on the sugar plantation in Hawaii. Some of my patients were hippies unaccustomed to bathing. Their body odors smelled strongly of fruits and vegetables, bearing witness to the fact that these individuals consumed a largely vegetarian diet. How could I expect otherwise? Characteristic odors of foods are carried into our bodies on our forks and spoons, and, naturally, what goes in . . . let's say it together . . . must come out.

Can't You Tell You Smell?

Dr. McDougall," Louise asked, "why does it seem most people are completely unaware of their own body odors? The vice principal where I teach emits visible fumes from her armpits. Any time one of us teachers is in her office, we gradually turn blue from holding our breath, and she hasn't a clue!"

"And why doesn't my boss notice when he hovers over my desk that I discreetly cover my nose to avoid inhaling his breakfast blend double-shot espresso breath?" added Larry.

I explained to the Bortons that most people are oblivious to their own body odors because of natural adaptations that occur within the nervous system. These adaptations cause us to quickly become accustomed to what is common. This *adaptive response* allows us to accept our familiar environment as "safe," and more importantly, clears our senses to recognize new and potentially dangerous stimuli—like those from a stranger's presence.

You've certainly had the experience of entering a person's home and quickly identifying unfamiliar scents, such as foods cooking on the stove, fresh paint, or the smell of a Christmas tree during the holidays. After a few minutes, you were no longer aware of these new odors—your nervous system had adapted. The same is true with body and breath odors. This is why I so quickly noticed the body odor of my hippie patients. Their vegetarian diet was very different from mine. A disturbing thought crossed my mind—What do *I* smell like, considering my usual fare of chicken, pork, beef, cheese, and eggs?

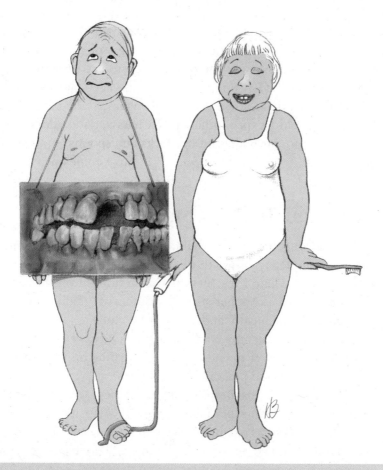

The mouth serves as a mirror reflecting the health of the rest of the body. Poor oral hygiene is one visible indication that overall health is ravaged with a plethora of serious diseases.

Two Brands of Bad Breath

There are basically two classifications of halitosis—*physiologic halitosis* (occurring in otherwise healthy people) and *pathologic halitosis* (occurring in the presence of disease). Pathologic halitosis in the mouth and nose areas can be caused by sinusitis, gum disease (gingivitis, periodontitis), an abscessed tooth, food impaction, or (as any parent of a three-year-old can attest) a foreign body lodged in the nose. Causes of halitosis from diseases that affect the rest of the system include kidney failure, liver failure, bowel obstruction, diabetes, and a metabolic condition known as fish-odor syndrome (trimethylaminuria).

Physiologic halitosis may be due to food and beverage consumption, alcohol and tobacco use, unclean dentures, or bacteria found in the mouth and other parts of the intestinal tract. Many foods can cause bad breath, the most commonly recognized culprits being garlic, onions, and certain spices that contain onion and garlic (such as curry and chili powders). However, the most common cause of offensive breath odor in otherwise healthy people is the release of sulfur compounds from foods commonly consumed in the Western diet.

Smell in an Eggshell

Larry wanted to know more about the sulfur compounds I mentioned that cause most cases of bad breath. I used an analogy to help them understand the process.

Just as the ingredients of a cake baking in the oven change form, sending delightful smells wafting throughout the house, so the process of proteins changing form within our bodies sends smells, often not so delightful, drifting from our mouths. In Scrabble-award-winning terms, this process is called *microbial putrefaction*. In layman's terms, bad breath is usually caused by bacteria breaking down proteins in the mouth and large intestine and the subsequent releasing of *gaseous sulfur compounds*, such as *dihydrogen sulfide* (H_2S) and *methyl mercaptan* (CH3SH).

Louise and Larry agreed that this did indeed sound like something that would stir up a stink.

Will the Real Sulfur Source Please Stand Up?

Next, of course, the Bortons wanted to know how to rid their diet of the sulfur sources.

They clearly understood, as Larry phrased it, "Reduce the amount of sulfur gases and you reduce the chance of offensive bad breath." This for Larry signified a world of romantic potential in the Borton household.

We've established that the most common cause of bad breath is the breaking down of proteins and the release of sulfur, which produces foul-smelling gaseous compounds. Of the twenty basic amino acids that make up all proteins in nature, only two contain sulfur: *methionine* and *cysteine*. So the equation is simple, a diet high in foods with sulfur-containing amino acids (methionine and cysteine), plus the body's natural bacterial breakdown process, equals chronic halitosis, affectionately known as "dragon breath."

"Dr. McDougall, please tell us cheeseburgers and pepperoni pizza have no stinking sulfur," pleaded Larry.

"Sorry, Larry. Red meats, poultry, cheeses, fish, shellfish, and all animal-derived foods are the ones with the most "'stinking sulfur,' as you so aptly put it."

Remember our formula for chronic halitosis? Well, here's another formula: a diet based on starches, vegetables, and fruits (without garlic and onions, which also contain generous amounts of sulfur), minus heavy intake of animal proteins, equals improved breath odor quality almost overnight.

> I shared with the Bortons the following comparisons of methionine (sulfur) content of food, based on calories consumed:
>
> - Beef contains four times more methionine than pinto beans.
> - Eggs contain four times more than corn.
> - Cheddar cheese has five times more than white potatoes.
> - Chicken contains seven times more than rice.
> - Tuna has twelve times more than sweet potatoes.

The Toothbrush Is Not Enough

Most of the foul odor we're speaking of is produced in the large intestine. Proteins are putrefied (broken down by bacteria) in the intestine, and then the sulfurous gases are absorbed through the intestinal wall into the blood stream, where they circulate until they reach the lungs and are eliminated through the breath. Since these odors originate from within, both toothbrushing and rinsing with mouthwash can only be expected to mask a small fraction of the offensive odors. The only way to achieve lasting fresh breath is to get at the root of the matter.

At the McDougall Health Center in Santa Rosa, California, we utilize a resort-style inpatient setting to introduce patients to the benefits of a plant-based diet and educate them about taking control of their own health. Patients consistently report the unexpected but pleasant benefit of fresher breath almost immediately upon starting our dietary program, and we have documented this change. Over a period of ten months, George Schneider, DDS, our investigative dentist, using a machine (Halimeter) that measures sulfur compounds in the patient's exhaled breath, found that the sulfur content in the patients' breath was cut in *half* after only seven days on our plant-based diet, absent of any animal products.

Reality Check Please: Your Personal Hygiene

Louise was quick to point out that people on TV and in the movies apparently do not suffer from bad breath. "They wake up in one another's arms with sunbeams dancing off their sparkling teeth, and lock lips in a passionate kiss as if devouring a ripe, juicy peach. Give me a break."

Larry continued, "Yeah, the truth is more like the TV ad for mouthwash where the couple wakes up, covers their mouths, and makes a mad dash for the bathroom to brush and rinse."

Larry and Louise are right. After changing the basic source of your unpleasant scents—your diet—there are still some matters of personal hygiene that need to be addressed.

Morning breath is most likely due to *anaerobic bacteria* throwing a reproductive party in a mouth that is closed for a great deal of the night during sleep. Because the bacteria involved in putrefaction and release of sulfur gasses prefer to live without oxygen, the closed mouth during sleep becomes their fertile breeding ground. Morning breath is a pungent example of the work of these unfriendly bacteria, most of which live on the back part of the top of the tongue.

Three Targets for Eliminating Bad Breath

1. To Rinse or Not to Rinse

About those mouthwashes that guarantee fresher, cleaner breath—don't get your hopes up. Most simply cover up odor and result in a temporary solution at best. However, studies show that a mouthwash containing zinc, chlorite anion, and chlorine dioxide directly oxidize gaseous sulfur compounds, taking the stink out of sulfur.

2. Scrub the Tongue

The tongue's surface is coated with dead and dying epithelial (skin) cells, blood cells, and bacteria. One of the simplest and most effective weapons in the fight against physiologic halitosis is regular tongue cleaning. In fact, cleaning the tongue is even more important than rinsing the mouth for eliminating unpleasant mouth odor. An infant toothbrush or a tongue scraper works best for this purpose.

3. See Your Dentist and Hygienist Now

Another area where odor-causing bacteria flourish is in the infection and inflammation of the gums and tissues surrounding the teeth in conditions such as gingivitis and pyorrhea. In order to remedy pathologic bad breath, leaking and broken fillings must be repaired. In addition, periodontal disease must be cured with meticulous flossing, a healthful plant-based diet, and visits to the dental hygienist every three to six months for thorough cleaning.

With regard to treatment of morning breath, a recent study showed that brushing the teeth or ingesting breath tablets (in this case, Breath Assure) had no influence on the sulfur gases, while eating breakfast and brushing the tongue resulted in strong trends toward decreased sulfur gases. In addition, rinsing with one teaspoon of hydrogen peroxide significantly reduced the concentration of sulfur gas for eight hours.

Halitosis and Health: An Undeniable Connection

Louise wasn't sure romantic potential was a potent enough motivator for giving up her evening snack of cheese and crackers. I assured her, "Bad breath isn't simply a cosmetic problem, because extremely low concentrations of sulfur compounds are also highly toxic to your body's tissues." These gases, especially methyl mercaptan, play a role in many serious physical diseases. They cause inflammation of the tissues surrounding and supporting the teeth, known as periodontitis. Periodontal disease has also been associated with other serious illnesses, including heart disease. Ingested sulfur causes inflammation of cells lining the intestinal tract (colitis) and occasionally a life-threatening condition known as ulcerative colitis. People with higher levels of the sulfur-based amino acid homocysteine in their bodies from eating a diet high in animal products have higher risks of heart attacks, strokes, deep vein thrombosis, Alzheimer's disease, and cancer. Fresher, cleaner breath is definitely a good thing, but the underlying improvement in health is indeed a powerful motivator for making dietary changes.

Food for Thought:
The Bortons Weigh In

After only a week on a plant-based diet, Larry and Louise reported positive outcomes from their new dietary choices. Larry said, "I didn't list bad breath as a medical complaint because I thought it was a normal thing I just had to live with. If I'd known the perks it could bring in the romance department, I'd have started this diet a long time ago."

Fresh breath was definitely an unexpected bonus for Larry and Louise, but even more positive changes would be forthcoming.

SUMMARY SHEET *from Dr. McDougall*

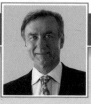

- *Your attractiveness to others depends upon your body odor.*

- *You can change your body odor and heighten your personal appeal almost overnight.*

- *The odor from sulfur smells like rotten eggs—undeniably unattractive.*

- *Animal food—meat, poultry, fish, shellfish, eggs, dairy products— are the main sulfur sources.*

- *Changing to a starch-based diet will reduce the amount of breath sulfur by one-half within a week.*

- *Garlic, onions, and strong spices impart lasting, sometimes unpleasant body odors.*

- *Avoid the use of tobacco, coffee, and alcohol for nontoxic breath.*

- *Use a tongue brush or scraper daily to remove odor-causing bacteria and debris.*

- *Floss and brush your teeth at least once daily to remove decaying remnants of food.*

- *The most effective mouthwashes contain chlorine dioxide.*

- *See your hygienist every three to six months for a thorough cleaning.*

- *See your dentist annually—more often if your teeth are in need of repair.*

CHAPTER 4

My Stomach's on Fire and I Can't Put It Out

Remember the old Pepto Bismol commercial where a visibly miserable man's belly blows up like a balloon as he bellows, "Indi——gestion," punctuated with a booming burp in the middle? This is how Larry and Louise described their routine post-dining experience. Larry kept a supply of antacid tablets on hand constantly, popping them like candy. Even in light of her other complaints, according to Louise this chronic indigestion was one of the biggest hindrances in her ability to enjoy life. "After all," she said, "what's the fun of gobbling down a scrumptious cheeseburger with all the trimmings when you know the price you're going to pay is a fireball in your chest?"

The Bortons are not alone. About 56 percent of people in Western countries report having experienced symptoms of indigestion at some point, while 36 percent report having symptoms at least once every four to six months. *Dyspepsia*, the clinical term for what is commonly referred to as indigestion or heartburn, causes such painful burning and discomfort in the upper abdominal region that patients like Larry and Louise report worse emotional well-being with indigestion than do people with heart failure, symptomatic heart disease, diabetes, and hypertension.

Based on my own experience with patients, I am convinced the problem of dyspepsia is even more common than is reported. Walk down the medication aisles of your local supermarket or drugstore and you'll see shelves of liquids and tablets intended to neutralize stomach acid and pills to prevent acid production. This class of medication, often referred to as *antiulcerants*, is the second leading category of prescription medication sold in the United States, with annual sales of nearly $11 billion and an average prescription cost of $109. Two antacids, Prilosec and Prevacid, ranked second and third in 2001 for raking in the largest sums of money spent on any prescription medication, with sales mounting to over $7 *billion* in the United States in that year alone—for just *two* medications. The Bortons, especially Larry, confessed to contributing significantly to the success of these drugs and a host of others in their search for relief from their nearly constant "indi———gestion."

GERD is the Word

D r. McDougall, why does it feel like someone's poured hot lava down my throat almost every time I eat?" Larry inquired. "It's almost enough to make me not want to eat. I guess you can tell by looking it hasn't actually stopped me yet."

I explained to Larry that like almost half of all cases of indigestion, his was most likely caused by the retrograde, or backward, flow of stomach contents up into the esophagus—a condition called *gastroesophageal reflux disease* or *GERD*. Because these stomach contents contain acids and other digestive juices, they can cause tissue damage and the resulting symptoms of discomfort. This condition is often described as a burning sensation behind the breastbone that radiates up toward the throat and is worsened by a meal or by lying down. Not surprisingly, these same feelings are often confused with those typical of a heart attack.

Diagnosis is usually made based upon the patient's description of symptoms. Further evaluation commonly includes looking into the esophagus through a tube known as an endoscope, although this extensive procedure (*gastroesophageal endoscopy*) fails to uncover evidence of disease in a significant percentage of people experiencing GERD symptoms. Larry and Louise were relieved to learn that I was not in a hurry to proceed with this sort of invasive investigation but that I could say with confidence that their indiges-

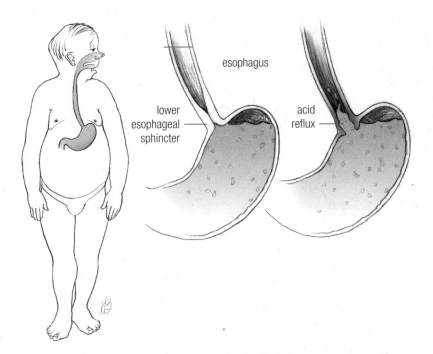

The control valve at the top of the stomach can become ineffective, allowing stomach acid to splash up into the esophagus. Acid burns everything it touches.

tion was due to GERD—a condition that could be dealt with in a simple, painless manner.

LES and Reflux

Louise was curious. "Why doesn't the stomach just contain the acid rather than spurting it back up into the esophagus? It's not supposed to work like that, is it?"

"Certainly not, Louise," I assured her. "The stomach only squirts acid back into the esophagus because of a malfunction of the *lower esophageal sphincter*."

"Huh?"

"The lower esophageal sphincter, we'll call it the LES, acts as a natural anti-reflux barrier, a gate if you will, at the opening between the stomach and esophagus. It relaxes when we swallow to allow food or liquid to pass through into the stomach and then returns immediately to a closed position. When the LES relaxes at inappropriate times, like between meals, harmful digestive acids flow back into the esophagus from the stomach, making us feel like someone's poured hot lava down our throats, as Larry mentioned earlier."

Causes of LES Dysfunction

Now that the Bortons understood the process of reflux, Larry wanted to know what he'd done to offend his LES and cause it to go on strike.

"There are two general reasons the LES may fail to function properly," I pointed out. "Structural damage from constipation, and temporary weakening—both related to . . ."

"Diet," chanted Larry and Louise simultaneously. They were beginning to get the message.

Constipation Does More Than Cause Worry

First let's look at the relationship between diet, constipation, and reflux. At least one well-respected researcher of gastrointestinal diseases from Yale University believes that more than 90 percent of GERD cases found in Western populations are a direct result of constipation. Severe straining to evacuate a hard, constipated stool causes the stomach to be pushed from its normal position in the abdominal cavity up into the chest. As a result of all that physical effort, the natural opening in the muscular diaphragm through which the esophagus passes is widened, creating a *hiatus (hiatal) hernia*. Eventually, part of the stomach lies in the chest cavity. With each inhalation of breath, negative pressures are exerted on the stomach, pulling acid up into the esophagus.

Extra pounds of abdominal fat can mechanically force the stomach into the chest cavity and its contents up into the esophagus. Restrictions caused by wearing tight clothing can produce similar effects. The immediate solution may be as simple as loosening your belt. Long-term relief of upward pressure on the stomach comes from permanent fat loss—best accomplished by following the same diet Larry and Louise are already adopting for their long list of intestinal troubles.

Larry bobbed his head emphatically, "That's me, Doc! So how do I get unstuck?"

I told him that one option would be to live with my colleague's mother who asked every other day as he was growing up, "Honey, have you had a bowel movement?" and dispensed generous doses of foul-tasting laxatives or, heaven forbid, an enema in response to an unfavorable reply. However, the healthier and more pleasant option would be to eat a diet rich in fiber and to avoid consumption of dairy products, which cause constipation by paralyzing the muscles of the bowels. Dietary fiber, which creates a bulkier, softer stool, is only present in plant foods. The meat-and-dairy-based, highly refined Western diet provides 8–14 grams of fiber daily, whereas a healthful diet based on starches, vegetables, and fruits packs a powerful 40–100 grams of dietary fiber. Mom was right. Eat your roughage.

Short-Term LES Dysfunction: Just a Bite Away

I n addition to long-term damage to the LES from years of constipation, there is also short-term (transient) LES dysfunction that occurs with consumption of certain foods. Most of these foods are believed to cause heartburn by decreasing the strength of the lower esophageal sphincter and increasing the number of relaxations of this sphincter. If you're like Larry and Louise and millions of others who consume the typical Western diet, what I have to share might not be welcome news. But, like Larry and Louise, you deserve to know which foods are making you miserable—even if they are your favorites—so that you can feel better. Grab a hankie. And remember, this is for your own good.

High-Fat Diet

As long as thirty years ago, a high-fat diet was recognized as a cause of acidity, heartburn, and belching. After a three-year period of observation, one doctor reported that a diet with no added fat cured 425 of 532 patients who were found to be fat-intolerant. More recently, studies at the University of Virginia Health Sciences Center confirmed that fat causes heartburn, with other research demonstrating that the reflux of acid back into the esophagus becomes progressively worse over the next three hours after eating a meal high in fat.

This same group of researchers from Virginia found another way to produce reflux. By inflating balloons that had been inserted in people's stomachs, the researchers produced an increase in the rate of LES relaxations. Adding their two findings together, their overall conclusion was that large fatty meals, which overdistend the stomach, are a major cause of heartburn. Did we really need researchers to tell us a supersized meal at Dottie's Deep-Fried Paradise equals a bad case of heartburn?

Coffee

Coffee (sorry, even decaf) causes indigestion by reducing LES function, though the effects of decaf are somewhat milder. Both regular and decaf cause the stomach to generate large amounts of acid—thus, chemicals in the coffee bean other than the caffeine itself are the acid-producing agents. However, recent studies suggest that LES dysfunction and gastroesophageal reflux, rather than acid production, are responsible for most of the heartburn symptoms caused by coffee. For relief, coffee drinkers must switch to beverages like herbal tea or one of the popular grain drinks rather than decaf. But the news isn't all bad for you lifelong java lovers—although there is considerably more indigestion among coffee drinkers, there is no increased risk of stomach or duodenal ulcers.

Cigarettes and Alcohol

Both cigarette smoking and alcohol can compromise LES function and cause indigestion. Most of the distress from alcoholic beverages comes from irritation of the stomach lining and the production of acid. Wine and beer cause much more stomach distress than do distilled spirits, like whiskey and vodka.

Onions

Onions significantly increase all measures of indigestion and have been found to be a potent and long-lasting cause of reflux in heartburn patients.

If you can't live without onions, no problem—simply cook them. Cooking onions destroys substances that are the cause of indigestion. The same holds true for green peppers, cucumbers, and radishes, which most often cause indigestion when consumed raw.

Chocolate

Chocolate syrup (even low-fat syrup) produces immediate and sustained decreases in LES pressure that can lead to symptomatic reflux. Approximately 40 percent of people surveyed had symptoms of heartburn after eating chocolate. Dark chocolate, with its high fat content (50 percent fat), may cause an even greater fall in LES pressure and more heartburn than regular chocolate.

Fruit Juices

Many people experience sour stomach and burning indigestion as a result of diluting citrus juices such as grapefruit or orange juice. Citrus fruits, as well as tomatoes and spicy foods cause most of their distress by direct irritation of the tissues of the esophagus and stomach rather than by lowering LES pressure. Surprisingly, acid is not the cause of heartburn from citrus foods, since neutralized orange juice also produces heartburn. In addition, whole fruit rarely causes digestive distress, so it is thought that the heartburn effects of fruit juice must somehow result from the disruption of the whole-fruit fibers and other protective substances in the process of turning fruit into juice.

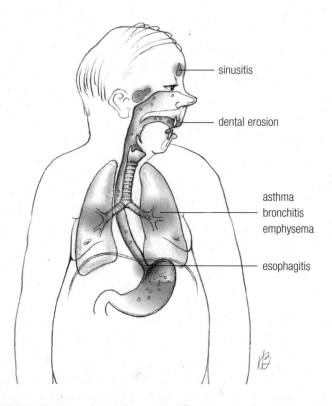

sinusitis

dental erosion

asthma
bronchitis
emphysema

esophagitis

Stomach acid is caustic to the tissues of the teeth, throat, sinuses, and lungs—
causing dental erosions, hoarseness, coughing, drainage, and asthma. Keep the
acid in your stomach with simple changes, especially a better diet.

Acid Damage from
the Teeth to the Lungs

You may be as shocked as the Bortons were to learn that the consequences of reflux extended beyond the pain and discomfort itself, as if that weren't enough. Gastroesophageal reflux disease can also cause conditions as serious as deep ulcers and cancer (adenocarcinoma of the esophagus), in addition to erosion of the teeth and even asthma.

In response to continuous reflux of stomach acids into the mouth, the enamel of the teeth breaks down (erodes), leaving permanent damage to this protective layer of the teeth. One study of individuals with dental erosions found that 83 percent had evidence of GERD. This relationship was confirmed when 40–70 percent of people with GERD were found to have erosions. The worse the reflux, the more likely that dental erosion has taken place.

Acid that is refluxed up into the back of the throat can then be inhaled into the bronchial (airway) tubes and burn them, causing constriction, swelling, and the production of large amounts of mucus. Between 34 and 89 percent of asthmatics have GERD, while 75 percent of children with asthma experience GERD. Patients with asthma caused by GERD commonly complain of heartburn, regurgitation, and difficulty swallowing, with worsening of symptoms following meals and after lying down. Even with the absence of reflux-related symptoms, following a healthful diet that reduces the chance of reflux, raising the head of the bed by four to six inches,

Reflux Causes Many Common Health Problems

DAMAGE TO THE MOUTH AND SINUSES

- Dental erosions
- Mouth ulcers
- Loss of taste
- Mouth pain
- Sinusitis
- Otitis media in children
- Ear pain and inflammation

DAMAGE TO AIRWAYS

- Asthma
- Chronic cough
- Bronchitis
- Emphysema
- Pneumonia
- Laryngitis
- Chronic hoarseness
- Throat inflammation
- Vocal cord ulcers
- Noncardiac chest pain

and using antacids (as a last resort) will help most people find relief from asthma, as well as many other breathing problems, and reduce their need for asthma medications.

Top Three Ways to Get Heartburn: And the Winners Are . . .

Knowing the Bortons' affinity for fast food, I decided to speak their language. I shared with them the findings of investigators looking into the causes of heartburn who took on the challenge of finding the top three meals guaranteed to cause indigestion. Their three winners (or losers, if you're on the heartburn-suffering end) were:

1. A *McDonald's Quarter Pounder,* a small order of fries, and an 8-ounce chocolate milkshake.

2. A *McDonald's Sausage Biscuit with Egg,* one slice of cheese, 30 grams of raw onion, and 8 ounces of Borden's Dutch Chocolate Milk.

3. An 8-ounce *Wendy's Chili* and 8 ounces of red wine (not from Wendy's, of course).

Given these results, it appears that the fast food industry and the antacid industry are a match made in heaven.

Medications for the Treatment of GERD

As a dues-paying member of our "pill for every problem" society, Larry asked, "How about the 'purple pill' and some of the other drugs I hear about all day on TV and in magazines? Can't I still take those?"

The answer for Larry and Louise is yes. However, because of their costs, side effects, and failure to address the root of the problem, medications should only be used as a last resort. They may help you feel better temporarily, but you remain sick nonetheless.

Medications May Be Causing Your LES Dysfunction

- Calcium channel blockers (blood pressure pills)
- Meperidine (Demerol)
- Morphine
- Dopamine
- Beta-adrenergic antagonists
- Diazepam (Valium)
- Barbiturates
- Theophylline (for asthma)
- Progesterone

There are several classes of medications that offer some relief from GERD and indigestion. Liquid and tablet antacids, H_2 receptor antagonists (see sidebar, below), and proton pump inhibitors all reduce the amount of acid in the stomach. Some agents, such as bethanecol (Edronax), increase the LES pressure, thereby reducing the incidence of reflux. Alginic acid (Protacid) forms a protective foam barrier, and sucralfate (Carafate) buffers some of the acid.

All medications can cause side effects, but the pills you swallow to stop the production of stomach acid are the most troublesome. H_2 receptor antagonists may cause mental changes,

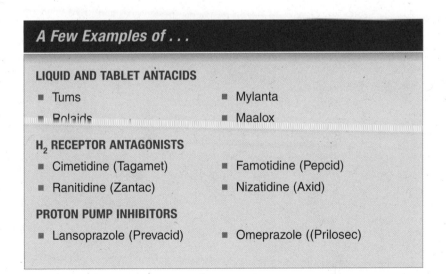

A Few Examples of . . .

LIQUID AND TABLET ANTACIDS

- Tums
- Rolaids
- Mylanta
- Maalox

H_2 RECEPTOR ANTAGONISTS

- Cimetidine (Tagamet)
- Ranitidine (Zantac)
- Famotidine (Pepcid)
- Nizatidine (Axid)

PROTON PUMP INHIBITORS

- Lansoprazole (Prevacid)
- Omeprazole ((Prilosec)

increased estrogen activity (which can cause enlarged breasts in men), and interference with the body's metabolism of other medications. In addition, there is some concern that H_2 receptor antagonists and proton pump inhibitors may cause stomach cancer with long-term use.

The Bortons Put Out the Flames

After our initial visit, Larry and Louise went home committed to following my recommendations—a diet based on cooked starches with the addition of fruits and vegetables. Looking for immediate relief, they kept their portions of raw food small, avoiding fruit juices, onions, green peppers, radishes, and cucumbers. Larry cut way back on his flaming Louisiana Hot Sauce. Results occurred almost immediately, and they were able to throw away their antacids. Larry even called to tell me how much he was enjoying his meals now that he didn't have a final course of heartburn to look forward to. Louise began trying new recipes and looking forward to cooking because she knew the reward would be a delicious meal with no painful price tag attached.

SUMMARY SHEET *from Dr. McDougall*

- *GERD results from an incompetent lower esophageal sphincter (LES). Years of unhealthful eating have caused sphincter malfunction.*
- *A plant-based diet, low in fat and high in fiber, is ideal for the health of this first part of the intestine—esophagus and stomach.*
- *People with very sensitive stomachs must avoid raw onions, green peppers, cucumbers, radishes, fruit juices, and hot spices.*
- *Eat small meals frequently to prevent overdistending your stomach and reduce the tendency to reflux.*
- *Lose weight if you are obese, and wear loose clothing to reduce reflux.*
- *Coffee, even decaf, is one of the most common causes of stomach distress.*
- *Decaffeinated coffee causes almost as much GERD and indigestion as regular—switch to water, cereal beverages, or herbal teas.*
- *Raise the head of the bed four to six inches to allow gravity to keep the contents in your stomach while prone (wedges specifically designed for elevating the upper body and extra pillows will not help—they only bend you at the middle).*
- *Stop all unnecessary medications that may be causing GERD and indigestion.*
- *Antacid medications should be used only as a last resort.*
- *Many health problems, from sinusitis to asthma, can be relieved by stopping acid reflux.*

CHAPTER 5

What's Eating You?

SAYING SO LONG TO ULCERS

After several months of healthful eating and feeling better than ever, Louise fell off the wagon, so to speak. With the holiday season came temptation in the form of fat-filled buffet tables, wine-and-cheese gatherings, and chocolate-covered everything. The post-smorgasbord consequences brought Louise to my office one crisp January morning.

"Dr. McDougall, for the past few weeks I've had the most horrible stomach pain. I'm worried it might be something really serious. I tried drinking milk like someone told me, but I just ended up with a bad bout of diarrhea. What's wrong with me?"

Louise came clean regarding her dietary indiscretions of the past festive month and admitted she'd been free of digestive problems until succumbing to the seduction of one party tray after another—straying far from the McDougall Diet recommendations. Her particular favorite was the ham roll-ups stuffed to overflowing with cream cheese. No wonder she was experiencing such distress.

Burning stomach pain was not a new symptom for Louise. Through the years she'd suffered bouts for which doctors had prescribed a variety of pills. The pain had become progressively worse over time, and this current flare-up was causing Louise considerable concern. Tests showed Louise was suffering from a duodenal ulcer, fortunately not yet at the point of bleeding. Stomach pain was Louise's notification of injury and her warning to make changes in

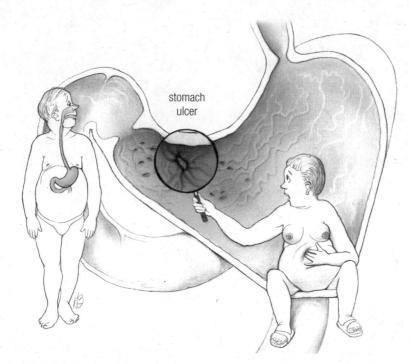

stomach
ulcer

Holes in your stomach are made by wrong choices at the dinner table and medications. Plus, unfriendly *H. Pylori* bacteria can make this organ their home, enhancing the damaging effects of meat, dairy, and NSAIDs.

order to avoid further damage. Armed with renewed motivation to return to a healthful diet, Louise needed the reinforcement of education to help her understand how the foods she had eaten all her life had contributed to this painful condition.

"Louise, your stomach is the first rest stop for everything you swallow—a one-quart vat that holds all the foods and beverages you consume. These contents may remain in the stomach for minutes or hours before moving on to the small intestine. The stomach's lining produces powerful enzymes and acids that break down the food before it's sent on through the digestive system."

"If these acids are so powerful, why don't they eat a hole right through the stomach, Dr. McDougall?"

"Good question, Louise. They certainly would if not for a protective mucous lining that acts as a barrier in the stomach and first part of the small intestine (the duodenum), keeping these acids and enzymes contained. However, as in your case, if this protective barrier breaks down, a sore commonly known as an ulcer develops in the stomach wall."

The stage was now set for Louise to learn about how food can affect the stomach, and about the stomach's ability to heal and to remain healthy.

Hurry, Worry, and Curry Cause What?

Quit your job, take two tranquilizers, and cut out spicy foods." Thirty years ago, this dictum would have summed up the advice given by well-meaning doctors, like myself, who learned in medical school that ulcers of the stomach and duodenum (also known as peptic ulcer disease) were due to "hurry, worry, and curry."

So convinced was the medical community of the "stress causes ulcers" theory that one of the commonly prescribed treatments for this serious condition was a surgical procedure called a *vagotomy*, in which the vagus nerve (the primary brain-stomach connection) was severed by the surgeon's scalpel. Treatments such as this have ceased to exist because they are brutal and simply do not work. Harmful foods, not harmful thoughts, cause ulcers and indigestion. The real surprise here is that the foods most people consider to be harmful to the stomach are not, and the so-called stomach-soothing foods are the ulcer-causing culprits!

Hot Doesn't Always Equal Harmful

Traditional wisdom has it that those hot, spicy condiments, like pepper or curry powder, burn holes in the stomach. Indeed, anyone who has enjoyed the ethnic enticements at a Thai, Mexican, Indian, or Szechwan Chinese restaurant will agree—they're called "hot" foods for a reason. In my early days as a doctor on a sugar plantation on the Big Island of Hawaii, my Korean patients frequently hurried to my office fanning their burning bottoms, a result of the previous evening's meal of *kimchi,* made from cabbage and hot chiles. Zesty spices, such as black pepper, chili powder, and red pepper, can indeed set you fanning from one end of the digestive tract to the other.

But despite their well-earned smoldering reputation, studies show that these spices do *not* typically injure the stomach's lining. In one study, eight men and four women were fed four different test meals and then twelve hours later underwent endoscopic examination (a tube passed into the stomach that allows direct visualization of the stomach's lining). Only two cases of injury were seen following the spicy meals—one with pepperoni pizza, the other with Mexican food containing an ounce of jalapeño chiles. By contrast, a bland meal *with* aspirin caused injury in eleven of the twelve participants, while the bland meal alone (no aspirin) caused no injury.

In a follow-up test, one ounce of freshly ground jalapeño chiles was placed *directly* into the stomach. Can you imagine the smoke coming from your ears if you had to *chew* and *swallow* that much pepper? Amazingly, twenty-four hours later, *no* visible stomach damage was seen.

More good news if you prefer the spicy side of life—additional investigations have found *no* difference in rates of inflammation of the stomach in heavy consumers of spice, and *no* difference in the rate of ulcer healing in those patients consuming large amounts of red pepper daily. And here's the clincher . . . in experiments on rats, capsaicin (the active ingredient in pepper) was actually found to *protect* the stomach mucosa from damage caused by alcohol or aspirin. With the addition of your favorite spices, healthful eating doesn't have to mean boring eating!

Milk to the Rescue? Not!

Remember Louise's comment that someone suggested she drink milk for her stomach pain? This was no random piece of advice but a belief rooted in medical folklore. Until recent years, this undisputed bit of medical knowledge meant patients were subjected to an ineffective and even harmful regimen of treatment for their stomach distress and ulcer disease.

In the early 1970s, at the time of my residency training, one of the popular diets I was instructed to use for peptic ulcer treatment was *The Sippy Diet*, consisting of antacids and half-and-half dairy creamer given alternately every other hour. When studies were finally performed to assess this therapy, researchers found no improvement of the patients' ulcer disease. Furthermore, there was one very serious drawback for this seemingly logical treatment. British and American patients treated for ulcer disease with this milk-antacid regimen suffered two to six times more heart attacks at the end of a year compared with those treated with the "regular" hospital diet. I suppose death by heart attack would indeed relieve the patient of his or her ulcer distress, but other alternatives are preferable.

This *Sippy Diet* and other similar dairy-based "cures" emerged despite information to the contrary. Over eighty years ago scientists reported that milk was a strong acid-producing stimulant that was slowly emptied out of the stomach. The combination of eggs and milk was found to produce an even higher level of acidity and to cause greater delay in emptying out of the stomach than milk alone. As you can well imagine, the longer corrosive acid sits in the stomach, the greater the chances of damage to the stomach lining in the form of ulcers and inflammation.

In the mid-1970s, about the same time I was learning of that medical marvel *The Sippy Diet*, researchers were studying the effect of various forms of milk on gastric-acid secretion. In five patients in remission from duodenal ulcer disease, as well as in five normal subjects, an eight-ounce glass of whole, low-fat, and nonfat milk each produced similar significant increases in acid secretion. The researchers concluded that because milk contains both protein and calcium, and each are stimulants of gastric-acid secretion, there is reason to question its frequent ingestion by patients with peptic ulcer. So much for the medically sound "milk cure" for ulcers.

Louise piped in about this time in our discussion. "Enough about what's *not* true, Dr. McDougall. What really *does* cause ulcers, and what can I do about it?"

The Hole Truth about Ulcers:
Animal Foods, Alcohol, and Drugs

H ere at the beginning of the twenty-first century, doctors finally have a more accurate idea about what causes ulcer disease and how to treat it effectively. Current focus is on three areas: acid production, medications (NSAIDs—nonsteroidal anti-inflammatory drugs), and bacteria (*H. pylori*). From Louise's history, I knew these were indeed the three primary factors contributing to the development of her stomach ulcer—acid production from the foods she ate, long-term use of anti-inflammatory drugs for arthritis pain, and bacterial activity that thrives in the presence of NSAIDs.

High Animal Protein Means High Acid

The primary job of stomach acid is to digest protein from your meals. So naturally, the more high-protein foods you eat, like meat, poultry, shellfish, fish, and cheese, the more acid your stomach produces and secretes. Gram for gram, animal protein produces more acid than an equivalent amount of plant protein. As a comparison, one study showed 30–40 percent less stomach acid production with soy protein than with beef protein. According to another large study, peptic ulcers occur more often with milk, meat, and bread consumption, as well as higher fat intake (including olive oil and vegetable fats). Consumption of vegetables, on the other hand, was associated with lower incidence of ulcers. Louise was not doing herself any favors by skipping the veggie platter and indulging in the ham roll-ups.

Alcohol and Acid

Before sharing with Louise about alcohol and acid production, knowing her tendency to celebrate any and all occasions (even returning a library book or getting the mail) with a glass of wine, I reminded her of the old adage, "Don't shoot the messenger." Alcoholic beverages do cause an increase in stomach acid. However, pure alcohol is not the problem here. You'll recall in the last chapter we discovered that regular and decaffeinated coffee produce similar amounts of stomach acid because other chemicals in the coffee bean rather than the caffeine are the acid-producing substances. The same is true for acid indigestion and alcoholic beverages—it's not the alcohol causing the trouble. The two acid-causing substances, maleic and succinic acid, produced in beer and wine during fermentation, are the acid-producing agents. These acids are removed during the distilling process that produces "hard" liquor. Of the various types of alcoholic beverages, champagne produces the highest level of stomach acid followed by wine, sherry, and beer. The least distressing are brandy and other hard spirits, such as whiskey and gin. Larry, who has been known to enjoy an after-dinner cognac or two, was happy to latch on to this bit of information.

Toxic Damage from Common Pain Killers (NSAIDs)

Nonsteroidal anti-inflammatory medications (NSAIDs) are taken by millions of people like Louise for relief of pain. Popular NSAIDs are aspirin, Motrin, Advil, and Naprosyn. About 15 percent of those who frequently use these drugs develop gastric or duodenal ulcers. Within ninety minutes of taking one or two tablets of aspirin, most individuals develop acute injury to the stomach lining consisting of bleeding and erosions. Once injured, the stomach acid eats into the tissues. Many patients are unable to continue taking NSAIDs due to drug-related stomach upset.

NSAIDs work by inhibiting small hormones called prostaglandins (such as cyclooxygenase-COX) involved in inflammation and pain. Long-standing NSAIDs, like Motrin or aspirin, inhibit the activity of two hormones, COX-1 and COX-2. Unlike these traditional NSAIDs, newly marketed COX-2 inhibitors, like Celebrex, Betrax, and Vioxx, selectively block *only* the COX-2 enzyme. This is significant because the COX-1 enzymes produce prostaglandins that provide the protective barrier for the stomach lining. By blocking the COX-2 enzyme but not the COX-1 enzyme, these drugs reduce damage to the esophagus and stomach, compared to traditional NSAIDs, while still providing pain relief. It is important to note, however, that COX-2 inhibitor NSAIDs pose a serious risk—they have been shown to increase the chance of heart attack by two to five times and are no more effective at relieving pain than aspirin or regular NSAIDs. Many brands of COX-2 inhibitors have been removed from the marketplace due to such serious side effects.

I assured Louise that once she began faithfully following my McDougall Diet recommendations, she would most likely be able to discontinue all of her anti-inflammatory drugs. After reviewing her eating habits for the past few months, Louise noted a definite pattern. When she was sticking closely to my dietary recommendations, she rarely had to take medication for her arthritis pain. Still more motivation to get back on the wagon and stay there. The effect of diet on arthritis and other such conditions is beyond the scope of our present discussion of digestive issues; however, most of my patients do find relief from joint pain, headaches, and other body aches once they begin adhering to my dietary suggestions.

Blame It on the Bacteria

In 1982, two physicians isolated the bacteria known as *Helicobacter pylori* (abbreviated *H. pylori*) from the stomach tissues of patients with *gastritis* (chronic inflammation of the stomach lining). Subsequently, these bacteria have been found living in the stomachs of most people with stomach and duodenal ulcer disease. In developed countries like the United States, an estimated 25–50 percent of people are infected with *H. pylori*, while in countries with widespread unsanitary conditions the incidence is as high as 70–90 percent. Most infections begin in childhood, and the bacteria appear to spread by way of the feces of infected persons. The common housefly may also be a vector for the spread of *H. pylori* bacteria. Although all individuals infected with *H. pylori* exhibit evidence of gastritis on examination by endoscopy, most have no symptoms.

Despite the fact that *H. pylori* bacteria are believed to be the chief cause of ulcer disease, more than 80 percent of infected people *never* develop an ulcer. It seems that *H. pylori* are simply innocent bystanders in most cases. So who are the unfortunate ones who fall prey to the damaging effects of *H. pylori*? What makes these bacteria lie dormant in some, while in others they compromise the defenses of the stomach lining and facilitate the development of ulcer disease?

We know, at least in part, the answers to these questions. People who take NSAIDs and are at the same time infected with *H. pylori* are at least sixty-one times more likely to develop ulcers of the stomach and/or duodenum than are those who are not infected and do not take NSAIDs. In addition, those suffering from malnutrition (actually *over*nutrition) caused by the typical Western diet are more likely to develop ulcers in the presence of *H. pylori*. Research has shown that a healthful diet including lots of fruits and vegetables loaded with vitamin C protects against infection with *H. pylori*. Interestingly, extracts from a variety of plants, such as garlic, thyme, and East African herbal plants, inhibit the growth of *H. pylori* in the test tube.

Antibiotics for Ulcers: A Temporary Fix

Standard medical treatment in the form of a "triple therapy" accelerates the healing of ulcers. This regimen includes two powerful antibiotics and a single antacid or bismuth compound. For example, one form of "triple therapy" consists of bismuth subsalicylate (262 mg), metronidazole (250 mg), and tetracycline (500 mg), all taken four times daily for fourteen days, and yields a cure rate for ulcers of 85–90 percent. Because there are serious risks and substantial costs from "triple therapy," I recommend this as a last resort when there is a clear indication that the benefits well outweigh the risks. (This benefit-risk ratio will have to be determined by you and your doctor.) This therapy rarely relieves common indigestion and therefore should not be prescribed to individuals with acid reflux (GERD) or other forms of acid indigestion who do not have ulcers. Unfortunately, eradication of the *H. pylori* bacteria through drug therapy is only temporary. Once the antibiotics are stopped, patients are likely to be re-exposed and reinfected. For these reasons, Louise decided that her most promising source of relief lay on her dinner plate rather than in a prescription bottle.

Whole Foods or Hole Foods: Louise Makes Her Choice

After learning how a diet plentiful in starches, vegetables, and fruits would aid in the healing of her stomach ulcer and help prevent further injury, Louise went home determined to make better food choices. As an added measure of assurance, she began eating lots of broccoli and broccoli sprouts, which researchers have found can act as potent antibiotic agents against *H. pylori*. She also enjoyed a glass of cabbage juice each day, an agent found to help heal ulcers and chronic gastritis. Louise made it her habit to ask before every meal or snack, "Is this a 'hole-healing' food or a 'hole-making' food?" Within weeks the report was just as I expected—no more "hole" foods, no more debilitating stomach pain.

SUMMARY SHEET *from Dr. McDougall*

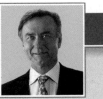

- *Ulcers are not caused by worry or any other kind of emotional distress.*

- *Damage to the stomach is due directly to its contents (foods, beverages, drugs, and bacteria).*

- *A plant-based diet, low in fat and high in fiber, gently soothes your stomach lining to good health.*

- *People with sensitive stomachs should avoid the few plant foods that cause indigestion, such as raw onions, green peppers, cucumbers, radishes, fruit juices, and hot spices.*

- *Spicy foods, like hot chiles, cayenne, and chili and curry powders, may cause a burning sensation, but rarely damage the stomach lining and never cause ulcers.*

- *Acid is produced by the stomach primarily to digest proteins like those found in meat, poultry, fish, milk, and cheeses.*

- *Reducing excess stomach acid means cutting way back on animal proteins.*

- *Milk and other dairy products increase stomach acid production and delay ulcer healing.*

- *Beer and wine contain acids—maleic and succinic—and are common causes of gastritis.*

- *NSAIDs (Motrin, aspirin, etc.) can be expected to damage the stomach and should be avoided whenever possible.*

- *H. Pylori bacteria, when combined with NSAIDs and unhealthful foods, commonly cause ulcers.*

- *Antibiotic therapy may be the last resort for ulcers, after attempting to gain relief through a healthful diet and discontinuation of ulcer-causing medications.*

- *Cruciferous vegetables (like broccoli and cabbage) and their juices may aid stomach healing.*

CHAPTER 6

Here's to a Happy Gallbladder

L ouise was the quintessential gallstone candidate—female, flatulent, (over) forty, and fat. So I wasn't surprised to see her in my office about a year and a half after our initial meeting complaining of nausea and severe stomach cramps. Louise had been doing very well following the McDougall Diet after a couple of start-stop attempts, but when her mother died, she began eating as a means of comfort. Rather than reaching for a soothing herbal tea, she drank soda and coffee by the potful. Instead of warm vegetable soup, she pulled out the oil and drowned her sorrow in deep-fried chicken and mashed potatoes swimming in butter. Succulent fresh fruits were replaced by cookies and pies with a hefty dollop of ice cream on top. Now Louise was paying the price.

Considering the eight hundred thousand hospitalizations and $5 billion spent annually on gallbladder disease, it's safe to say that a lot of folks are paying the same price. Over twenty million people in the United States harbor gallstones (that's 15 percent of the country's population), including half of all women over the age of seventy.

Women are almost twice as likely as men to develop gallstones. This is due in part to the presence of estrogen, which promotes the secretion of cholesterol into the bile. Not surprisingly then, hormone replacement therapy (HRT) for menopause, birth control pills, and the later months of pregnancy are associated with a further increase in the risk of gallstone formation.

Weight is also a risk factor for gallstone formation. Overweight people consume more food and cholesterol. Their bodies also make more cholesterol. The more overweight the individual, the greater the amount of cholesterol that is secreted into the bile. And finally, aging also results in increased cholesterol secretion by the liver, supersaturating the bile, which explains why gallstones occur four to ten times more frequently in older populations.

Despite the prevalence of gallbladder disease, few people know much about this tiny organ—how it functions or how to keep it healthy. These are the matters I discussed with Louise.

What Is the Gallbladder Anyway?

Louise's response upon learning that the problem was with her gallbladder echoed the sentiment of many patients I've encountered. She asked, "Dr. McDougall, what the heck does a gallbladder do anyway? They yank them out at the drop of a hat, so they must not be very important." Thus began Louise's education on the nature and function of the gallbladder.

True to its name, the gallbladder is quite simply a bladder, or sack, that collects gall, the yellowish-green bile produced by the liver. Once the bile is produced, it is diverted to this small, pear-shaped sack attached to the underside of the liver, where it is stored between meals. Soon after we finish eating, the gallbladder contracts, and the collected contents (bile) squirt into the intestine, mixing with and digesting fats and other food components.

Under Attack

Louise questioned, "Exactly why is my gallbladder attacking me? Did I do something to make it mad?" I continued with my explanation rather than pointing out that, yes, in fact, Louise's gallbladder was aggravated by what she was eating and that she could play a key role in appeasing its anger. We would get to that later.

When the cystic duct, which carries bile from the gallbladder to the small intestine, becomes blocked, or obstructed, the resulting symptoms are referred to as a gallbladder attack. During an attack, most patients experience pain in the mid-upper or right-upper sec-

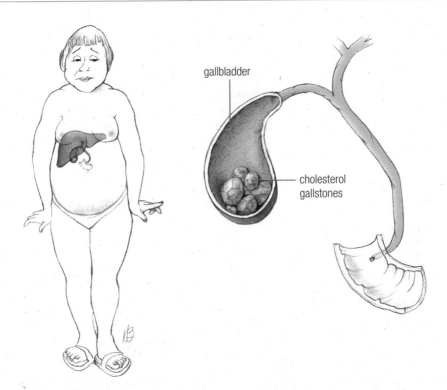

gallbladder

cholesterol gallstones

Gallstones, made of cholesterol, are so common in women, middle-aged and beyond, that they are almost "normal." That is, "normal" for people eating a high-fat, high-cholesterol diet.

tion of the abdomen, often radiating to the right shoulder blade. The pain is usually severe and steady, lasting from fifteen minutes to six hours, and often occurs at night, unrelated to meals. Nausea and vomiting are also common, symptoms that were right in line with Louise's presenting complaints. After the first attack, the probability of a second attack is between 50 and 70 percent within two years *if* there is no change in diet.

When the obstruction of the flow of bile is prolonged (more than six hours), distention and inflammation can develop, along with a secondary bacterial infection in about 50 percent of cases. This is a serious complication that usually requires immediate medical attention. Stones can also block the ducts draining the pancreas, causing pancreatitis.

Diagnosis of gallstones is usually made by ultrasound examination (sound waves penetrate the abdomen and pinpoint stones). This test can detect, painlessly and safely (without harmful radiation), 95 percent of stones larger than 2 mm (the size of a rice grain). Louise was surprised at how simple and painless the procedure turned out to be.

The Prescription for Gallstones

I f there were a recipe for gallstones, it would be this—eat lots of cholesterol. Remember, cholesterol is only found in animal products. Overconsumption of cholesterol is the primary cause of supersaturation of the bile and the resulting gallstones. Bile that is held in the gallbladder consists of various substances, including salts, electrolytes, bilirubin (a blood pigment), fats, drugs, waste products, and cholesterol. This cholesterol comes from the foods we eat as well as the cholesterol our bodies make. When the liver secretes an excess of cholesterol, the bile becomes supersaturated with this cholesterol and crystals begin to form that develop into rock-hard formations commonly referred to as gallstones (clinically termed cholelithiasis). Increasing the amounts of both saturated fat and cholesterol in the diet—in simple terms, the amount of animal-derived foods—supersaturates the bile. Over 90 percent of gallstones found in Americans are considered *cholesterol gallstones;* that is, consisting of 70–90 percent cholesterol by weight.

Dietary fiber plays a key role in preventing gallstones. (Only plants contain fiber.) A low-fiber diet results in remnants of food moving through the large intestine at a slowed rate. This sluggish movement of bowel contents allows for more absorption of one form of bile acid (deoxycholic acid) that raises the risk of stone formation. A high-fiber diet, by contrast, speeds the movement of bowel contents, limiting the absorption of this stone-forming bile acid.

You will find it interesting to know that no other animal besides the human is known to spontaneously develop cholesterol gallstones. This is because we eat a diet unnatural to our design and needs. The

Consider the following observations regarding the link between diet and gallbladder health:

1. Worldwide, there is a positive correlation between the amount of fat consumed and the incidence of gallstones in a population. Gallstones are rare in African and Asian countries.

2. American Indians, who have recently adopted the standard American diet, have a very high incidence of gallbladder disease; for example, 70 percent of Pima Indian women over twenty-five years of age suffer from gallstones. Tarahumara Indians of northern Mexico (genetically related to the Pima) follow their native diet of corn, beans, and squash and are essentially free of gallbladder disease.

3. Since World War II, the Western European diet has become richer in fat and cholesterol, and the incidence of gallstones has increased proportionally.

4. Prior to World War II, cholesterol gallstones were rare in Japan. With the Westernization of the Japanese diet, gallstones are becoming commonplace.

5. Vegetarians rarely develop gallstones.

typical Western diet based on meat, dairy, eggs, and refined foods is an aberration—consumed by a few kings, queens, and aristocrats of old, and only for the past century by many persons. It's no wonder then that Americans suffer such a high rate of gallbladder illness.

Weight Loss and Gallstones

Ironically, the overweight person who determines to improve his or her health by losing weight can end up with gallstones as a result of dieting. Within sixteen weeks of beginning a low-calorie diet, about 10 percent of dieters develop gallstones, and more than 30 percent develop gallstones within twelve to eighteen months following gastric bypass surgery (an extreme weight-loss measure).

How does weight loss lead to gallstones? When the body begins to shed pounds, stored cholesterol is released in large amounts from the body fat into the bloodstream and is then secreted into the bile. As a result the bile becomes supersaturated with cholesterol, the primary cause of gallstones.

Gallstones are more likely to occur under the following conditions during intentional weight loss:

1. The individual is obese upon beginning the diet.
2. The loss of weight is greater than 24 percent of initial body weight.
3. The rate of weight loss is greater than 1.5 kg (3 pounds) per week.
4. The diet is very low in calories with little fat.
5. The person started with a high serum triglyceride level.

How Can I Win if I'm Losing?

Louise immediately jumped to the conclusion that her previous attempts at losing weight were at the root of her present gallbladder troubles. She asked, "Is it safe to follow the McDougall Diet and lose weight?"

I assured her, "It *is possible* to lose weight without developing gallstones. This complication of gallstone formation has been seen mostly after surgery performed for weight loss and with very low calorie diets (like liquid diets). Over the past twenty-five years, out of the thousands of individuals who've lost weight with the McDougall Program, fewer than a dozen have developed gall-stones—far less than the 10 percent predicted by studies of other weight-loss programs. Because our recommended diet contains no cholesterol and is high in fiber, participants lose an average of 3.5–4.5 pounds a week, without the risk of supersaturation inherent with most other diets. By following our recommendation to eat until they are fully satisfied, our participants keep their weight loss at a safe level and avoid an angry gallbladder from supersaturation of cholesterol in the bile."

I concluded our conversation with a gentle reminder: "Louise, the foundation for your present health has been laid for decades with one high-fat, high-cholesterol meal after another. The start-stop approach to healthful eating has unfortunately caused some setbacks in the process of regaining your health. You can be certain the consistent type of healthful eating I'm prescribing will *not* aggravate or cause further gallstones."

Choosing Your Strategy for Gallstones You Now Own

As with most of my patients, I recommended to Louise a course of "expectant management" in lieu of aggressive treatment (immediate surgery), because her stones were not causing her any discomfort as long as she ate low-fat, McDougall-style fare. Once diagnosed with gallstones, only 10 percent of patients develop symptoms within the first five years and 20 percent within the first twenty years. This means a person with gallstones has an 80 percent chance of remaining asymptomatic (having no symptoms). Gallstones that don't hurt should be left alone. Scientific research clearly and consistently shows that the risk of death and disability is much greater with immediate surgery than with "expectant management," as long as the stones are not troublesome.

When symptoms do arise, the time-honored treatment of a low-fat diet will often alleviate the pain of gallbladder disease, thereby eliminating the need for surgical intervention.

Immediate Surgery

Patients with recurrent attacks that cannot be prevented are generally referred for cholecystectomy, a surgical procedure in which the gallbladder is removed through a four- to eight-inch incision in the abdomen. A less invasive form of this surgery, laparoscopic cholecystectomy, utilizes a small scope through which the gallbladder is removed, resulting in smaller scars and quicker recovery than with "open" surgery. The number of surgeries in the United States has increased from 500,000 annually in 1987 to 770,000 in 1996, largely because of this new, "easier" procedure. Therefore, many patients with questionable indications are undergoing surgery for gallbladder removal.

Doctors have been known to coerce patients into surgery with the threat that their gallstones can lead to gallbladder cancer. Although this may be true, the risk is extremely small (one in one hundred thousand for the United States) and should never be used as a reason for surgery. Patients are told that obstruction by a stone may occur and require emergency surgery. True again, but when all risks are averaged, the patient is still better off delaying surgery and leaving his or her gallbladder intact.

Patient surveys two to twenty-four months following either open surgery or laparoscopic cholecystectomy indicate that 80–90 percent of patients regard the operation as highly successful. However, 40–50 percent of patients still report having one or two remaining symptoms, such as abdominal discomfort from excess bowel gas or dull pain.

Why Keep Your Gallbladder?

Louise wanted to weigh all the facts before making her decision regarding aggressive surgical treatment versus my "expectant management" recommendation. "Dr. McDougall," she asked, "other than the risk of surgery itself, is there any other reason I should keep my gallbladder?" Louise spoke for countless others similarly grappling with this decision.

"Louise," I said, "I certainly understand your thinking. Because of the tendency to remove the gallbladder at the slightest sign of symptoms, we have come to believe that this organ must play no significant role in our health. This assumption is simply untrue."

I went on to explain that the purpose of the gallbladder is to store the greenish fluid called bile that is continuously synthesized by the liver. When you eat, the gallbladder contracts, emptying its contents into the small intestine, where the bile mixes with the food. If there is no storage sack (gallbladder), then the bile constantly drips into the intestine even when no food is present. In this concentrated form, bile acids are very irritating to the lining of the intestine, often causing diarrhea—a very common complaint after gallbladder removal. This irritation of the intestine can ultimately lead to intestinal cancer, as indicated by the higher incidence of cancer of the right side of the colon in those who have undergone this surgery.

For these reasons (diarrhea and cancer), it is important for people without their gallbladder to make wise food choices. Since fat is the primary stimulus for bile acid production, by eating a low-fat, high-fiber diet, individuals can often eliminate or drastically reduce the side effects of living without a gallbladder. Dietary fiber (which is only present in plant foods) will combine with and deactivate bile acids, thus protecting the bowel. If this change in diet fails to relieve diarrhea, the next step in treatment is to use a "bile acid sequestering agent," such as activated charcoal or doctor-prescribed cholestyramine (Questran) or colestipol (Colestid).

"So, Louise," I concluded, "despite the medical community's enthusiasm for aggressive gallbladder treatment, even to the extent of yanking out a marginally symptomatic organ, the best thing you can do is to keep your gallbladder and keep it healthy. Besides keeping bile properly contained, this little sack may save your life by screaming in agony whenever you eat fatty foods. If you pay attention and heed its warning, your suffering gallbladder could help you prevent heart disease, strokes, and even cancer. And it may prove to be the most effective weight-loss aid you could ever wish for by forcing you to choose wisely at the dinner table."

What About Dissolving Gallstones?

Like most folks with gallstones, Louise just wanted them gone—out of her body. She inquired, "I've heard there's some way of dissolving gallstones. Why can't we just do that and I'll be rid of them for good?" I went on to explain Louise's available options.

"You're right, Louise. Two bile acids, chenodeoxycholic acid (CDCA) and ursodeoxycholic acid (UDCA), when given as medications, have been found to dissolve gallstones. A combination of CDCA with UDCA has about a 50 percent success rate in completely dissolving noncalcified stones within six months of therapy. You may have heard of Actigall, a common prescription form of UDCA. Actigall is a bile-acid medication that's also used to prevent gallstones in people on rapid-weight-loss diets. Actigall is most effective if the gallstones are small or "floatable" (high in cholesterol). If the gallbladder isn't functioning properly, the Actigall won't work."

"So am I a candidate for Actigall, Dr. McDougall? Are my stones 'floatable'?"

"Yes, you are, Louise. With the addition of cholesterol-lowering medications, such as lovastatin (Mevacor) and simvastatin (Zocor), that lower both serum and bile cholesterol, the Actigall therapy can be even more effective. A low-fat diet has similar benefits, helping Actigall dissolve stones. But . . ."

"I knew there'd be a big but at the end. There always is."

"But, Louise, the problem with Actigall therapy alone is that the gallstones soon return. The reason is obvious—unless the diet is changed to avoid supersaturating the bile with cholesterol at every meal, gallstones will form again. The good news is that evidence to date indicates that the same low-fat, no-cholesterol diet that prevents initial stone formation will also prevent recurrences of stones once they are dissolved using a medication like Actigall."

"So, what would you do, Dr. McDougall, if it were your stones and your gallbladder?"

"If it were me, Louise, I'd keep my stones and my gallbladder. Once your gallbladder symptoms are relieved by following a low-fat, no-cholesterol diet, we will simply resume our plan of "expectant management." Why undergo surgery or take a medication like Actigall that carries its own possible side effects when you can most likely alleviate your symptoms with simple, low-cost, completely free-of-side-effects dietary changes. I've seen it over and over in my patients—when you eat well, your gallbladder stays well."

Does Louise Keep Her Gallbladder?

After talking it over with Larry, Louise chose to follow my recommendation of "expectant management." Having experienced firsthand the improvement in health that accompanied her adherence to the McDougall Diet, Louise was hopeful that she could appease her angry gallbladder by following this same plan—this time for good! I was confident that she would not only calm her agitated gallbladder, but also lose weight and feel fantastic in the process, if she would make the dietary changes I prescribed. Only time would tell if she was willing to stick with the diet and reap the rewards.

SUMMARY SHEET *from Dr. McDougall*

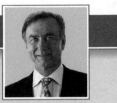

- *The gallbladder is an important storage sack used to collect bile from the liver between meals.*
- *Gallbladder disease and accompanying gallstones are caused by the rich Western diet.*
- *Supersaturation of the bile with cholesterol is the hallmark for gallstone formation.*
- *More than 90 percent of gallstones are made primarily of cholesterol.*
- *Female gender, obesity, elevated body estrogens from various sources, and age are associated with a greater chance of gallstones.*
- *Gallstones plague 15–50 percent of the American population.*
- *Painful attacks occur when stones plug the outlet ducts from the gallbladder and liver.*
- *Rapid weight loss may cause the movement of cholesterol from the body fat to the gallbladder, increasing the risk of stones.*
- *Stones that are presently causing no symptoms (pain) should be left alone.*
- *A low-fat diet can alleviate gallbladder pain in most cases.*
- *The threat of gallbladder cancer and emergency surgery should not be used to scare a patient into submitting to surgery.*
- *Many people still suffer from abdominal distress even after gallbladder removal, often because they still have not changed their diet.*
- *After losing the gallbladder, patients commonly have diarrhea and a higher risk of colon cancer.*
- *A plant-based diet eliminates postoperative diarrhea and reduces cancer risks.*
- *Gallstones can be dissolved with Actigall, but usually there is no reason to take this medication.*
- *A diseased gallbladder can serve a valuable purpose by reminding those who have excruciating pain to choose well at the dinner table.*

CHAPTER 7

The Liver
to the Rescue

Generally a fairly mild-mannered fellow, Larry Borton often metamorphosed into quite the party guy at his and Louise's weekly bowling night—with the help of a few beers, that is. Louise didn't seem to mind, but did request that he refrain from doing his Elvis impression when it was her turn to bowl. The Bortons usually enjoyed a nightly indulgence of some sort—usually a glass of wine or beer, and on occasion, Larry's favorite—an after-dinner cognac. Though neither showed signs of alcohol dependence, I felt it important to talk with them about how their regular use of alcohol could be harming their liver.

A rather portly individual, Larry's ears perked up when I told them that his diet may be as hard on his liver as his drinking—obesity, on rare occasions, encourages the progression of liver disease to a chronic, often fatal condition known as cirrhosis. I explained what the liver does and how alcohol, as well as certain types of food and other substances, can affect its ability to function properly. Larry was stunned to learn that his liver did more than just eliminate the inebriating effects of his bowling night beers.

The Great Detoxifier

The liver is the body's largest internal organ. It simultaneously synthesizes and breaks down dietary proteins, fats, and carbohydrates, and it regulates cholesterol and triglycerides. The

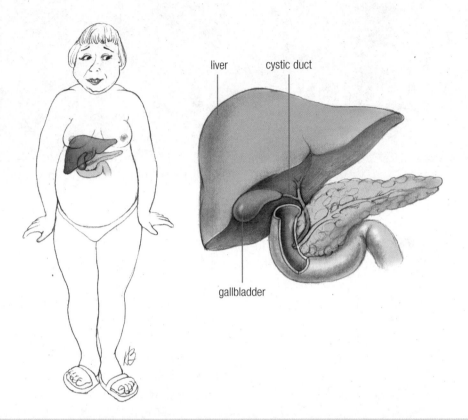

liver   cystic duct

gallbladder

You only have one liver, so expose your body to as few toxins as possible by eating a clean diet and avoiding alcohol, chemicals, medications, and infections.

liver is also the primary site for activation, clearance, detoxification, and excretion of most medications, drugs, and toxins that enter our body. In an effort to go easy on the liver, it is particularly important to avoid toxic substances, the most widely consumed, of course, being alcohol.

Chronic liver disease is the tenth leading cause of death in the United States, resulting in about twenty-five thousand deaths per year. Fortunately for those of us looking for salvation after years of abusing our bodies, the liver has a tremendous capacity to regenerate itself, even after serious injuries.

Foods the Liver Loves

During my basic medical training more than thirty years ago, I learned that the best diet for all liver ailments, from acute hepatitis to chronic liver failure, is a high-carbohydrate, low-fat, and low-protein diet. Carbohydrates are the energy sources most easily utilized by the liver. Carbohydrates also increase the production of insulin, which helps remove potentially toxic proteins from the body. There is evidence that carbohydrate intake lowers the risk of cirrhosis (a chronic, often fatal liver condition), whereas saturated fat intake significantly increases the risk associated with alcohol consumption. In addition, a high-carbohydrate diet limits the intake of proteins, which the liver must process.

Dietary protein can cause a person with liver failure to suffer further complications of his or her illness. During liver failure, protein degradation products become toxic to the body. When amino acids and other protein-breakdown products accumulate, encephalopathy (mental dysfunction) and hepatic coma often result. Vegetable protein is more easily tolerated than protein from animal sources by a person with impaired liver function. In fact, people with severe liver disease have been effectively treated by a diet that substitutes animal protein with vegetable protein as a single therapy—relieving encephalopathy and hepatic coma.

Fatty Liver Disease

Looking over Larry's recent lab tests I noticed elevated levels of enzymes from his liver. "Does that mean no more beer on bowling night?" Larry inquired with bated breath.

"Larry, my guess is these elevated levels are probably due to fat accumulation in your liver rather than to the effects of alcohol."

Larry was relieved but wanted to know what in the world I meant by fat accumulation. "You mean even my liver is fat?" With that began our discussion of Liver 101.

Fatty infiltration of the liver, medically termed *nonalcoholic steatohepatitis*, occurs when fats accumulate within the liver tissue. This fatty liver disease can lead to serious consequences, including inflammation, scar tissue formation (fibrosis), and cirrhosis. Autopsy reports indicate that 10–51 percent of people following the Western diet have moderate to severe accumulation of fat in the liver, and I suspect these numbers will be rising with the increasing epidemic of obesity. This condition is most commonly seen in people who are alcoholic, obese, diabetic, and/or have elevated triglycerides (hypertriglyceridemia). About 75 percent of affected individuals are women, and between 70 and 100 percent are obese.

As in Larry's case, fatty infiltration of the liver is usually discovered when routine blood tests, known as *alanine aminotransferase* (ALT) and *gamma glutamyl transferase* (GGT), reveal elevation of one or more of the liver enzymes. Other causes for elevation of these liver enzymes, such as heavy alcohol intake or viral hepatitis, must be ruled out before a diagnosis of nonalcoholic steatohepatitis can be determined. About half of these patients complain of fatigue and/or upper abdominal discomfort, while the other half report no symptoms.

High fat and oil consumption are associated with an elevation in liver enzymes. Most importantly, studies show that a ten- to fifteen-pound weight loss through healthful eating and exercise is a very effective means of healing the liver. Results can be seen in lower liver enzyme levels and in the disappearance of fat from the liver tissues on direct examination through biopsy (an invasive procedure that I do not recommend).

"So, Larry," I said, "if you will focus your attention on your diet, I predict that in no time at all your liver enzyme levels will be back to normal." I added, "Just to be safe, however, we also need to rule out the possibility that these liver abnormalities could be due to an infection, specifically hepatitis or a medication you might be taking."

Infectious Hepatitis

Hepatitis (inflammation of the liver) is usually due to a viral infection, but it can also be caused by medications and other chemical toxins. Viral hepatitis is commonly classified as A, B, and C, as well as by other letters. These viruses are spread by close contact with infected people or their body fluids (saliva, blood, and semen). Hepatitis B and C are almost always associated with illicit drug use, blood transfusions, and/or sexual contact. Hepatitis A is spread by the fecal-oral route, often through food or drink. Fortunately, there are effective vaccines for hepatitis A and B that greatly reduce the chance of infection.

Once infected, the body mounts a defense that attempts to eliminate the virus. However, in some cases this fails and the infection becomes chronic. Between 75 and 80 percent of those infected with hepatitis C go on to develop a chronic form of the illness, with more than 25 percent developing cirrhosis within forty years. Chronic infections from hepatitis B and hepatitis C viruses are major risk factors for most primary liver cancer cases worldwide.

I have personally encountered individuals who were able to reverse chronic viral hepatitis simply by changing to a low-fat, pure vegetarian diet, although at this time there is no published research to support such a claim. While the mechanism of this reversal is open to more research, it certainly makes sense that a healthier body through more healthful eating would enable the body's systems to mount a more formidable attack against any viral infection.

Herbs for Hepatitis

Herbal treatments for chronic hepatitis are highly effective and virtually free of side effects. For example, one of the earliest and most encouraging reports was published in 1988 in the *Lancet* medical journal. In this preliminary study, thirty-seven chronically infected patients were treated with a preparation of the plant *Phyllanthus amarus* for thirty days. When tested fifteen to twenty days following treatment, twenty two of the thirty seven patients (59 percent) had lost the hepatitis B surface antigen, the protein coat of the virus that indicates continued infection. By comparison, only one of twenty-three (4 percent) placebo-treated control subjects had lost the surface antigen. Some subjects were followed for up to nine months, and in no case did evidence of the chronic virus infection return. In addition, there were no serious adverse effects from the treatment. Recent reviews of the use of this herb have similarly concluded its significant effectiveness. Other herbal treatments, such as the Chinese *Jianpi*

Wenshen recipe and the Japanese herbal medicine *Sho-saiko-to,* have reportedly been effective in the treatment of infectious hepatitis.

The most commonly used herb for liver disease, including mushroom poisoning, alcoholic liver disease, and viral hepatitis, is milk thistle. It appears to protect the liver cells against a variety of toxins, as well as help detoxify the liver and promote regeneration of liver cells. Other herbs, including *Picrorhiza kurroa, Curcuma longa* (turmeric), *Camellia sinensis* (green tea), and *Glycyrrhiza glabra* (licorice), have also been used to promote liver health.

Sadly, due to the nature of the pharmaceutical and medical industries, patients and even doctors are rarely apprised of the benefits of herbal therapies. Both patients and doctors are very well aware, however, of the latest drug therapies. The best standard medical treatments for chronic hepatitis are with drugs known as interferon and ribavirin. These medications offer about a 40 percent chance of eliminating chronic liver infection. The costs are high— forty-eight weeks of interferon/ribavirin combination therapy should cost approximately $10,000. Besides monetary cost, these treatments often cause very serious side effects.

Avoid Liver-Toxic Chemicals

The list of occupational and environmental chemicals (like carbon tetrachloride) that are known to cause liver damage is too extensive to provide here. Two food-derived toxins suspected of causing liver cancer are nitrosamines (found in preserved meats, such as luncheon meats and hot dogs) and aflatoxins (found in moldy grain and peanut products). Following alcohol and high fat consumption, prescription and over-the-counter drugs are the most frequent causes of liver damage.

You Only Get One Liver

After further testing, I was able to reassure Larry that his elevated enzyme levels were not due to hepatitis or to any medication he was taking. The choice was then his to make.

Commonly Encountered Liver-Toxic Drugs

NSAIDs (Advil, Motrin, etc.)

COX-2 inhibitors (like Celebrex and Vioxx)

Painkillers (Tylenol)

Cholesterol-lowering drugs (like Mevacor, Zocor, Lipitor, and niacin)

Diabetic medications (Precose, Actos, Avandia, and sulfonylureas)

Estrogens

Anabolic steroids

Antibiotics

Antifungals

Anticonvulsants

Antidepressants

Antiarthritic (methotrexate)

Anti-acne (Accutane)

Vitamin A (retinol)

For a more complete listing of drugs that can cause liver damage, look through a *Physicians' Desk Reference* at your local library or bookstore.

He pledged to change his diet—to give up beer on bowling night (at least a couple of times a month), to eat low-fat, high-carbohydrate foods, to make every attempt to avoid prescription drugs, and to be careful with any household chemicals. He knew the cost of damaging his liver was just too great to take any more risks. I was hopeful that this would be motivation enough for Larry to keep his pledge.

Chapter Seven

SUMMARY SHEET *from Dr. McDougall*

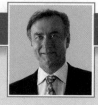

- The liver detoxifies internally produced and externally derived substances and is sometimes injured in the process.

- A high-carbohydrate diet, low in fat and protein, is the preferred fuel for the liver.

- Alcohol is the most common toxin injuring the liver.

- Fatty infiltration of the liver is a serious condition caused by the rich Western diet.

- The liver has an astonishing capacity to recover—after the removal of injurious substances like alcohol and fat.

- Infectious hepatitis is commonly caused by viruses, but the risk of transmission can be reduced by immunization with hepatitis A and B vaccines.

- Various herbal preparations offer hope for patients chronically infected with viral hepatitis.

- Interferon/ribavirin therapy, prescribed by doctors, may be beneficial, but it also entails significant cost and potentially serious side effects.

- Medications and environmental chemicals can cause serious liver damage—be careful.

CHAPTER 8

In Search of the Perfect Bowel Movement

When last we saw Louise she was determined to get back on track with her healthful eating habits in order to keep her gallbladder. On our next visit, I was thrilled to hear how well she'd done with cutting out fats and eating more fruits and vegetables. I was also thrilled to see her walk through the door with Larry. Though Larry and Louise had both followed the McDougall Diet in fits and starts since our first meeting, Larry's experience was characterized more by the fits than the starts, and he was experiencing a multitude of digestive difficulties. Louise was also experiencing some troubling symptoms of her own, which we'll talk about in our next chapter.

After one of Larry's painful, prolonged visits to the bathroom, Louise had suggested he come with her to her next appointment, "just to check in with Dr. McDougall." He consented because, as he admitted to me that day, "Dr. McDougall, I'm fed up with making a career out of going to the bathroom." With that comment, Larry unknowingly launched us into an enlightening discussion of all things bowel-related.

Only those precious grandmotherly types who delight in recounting frequency, color, and consistency find a discussion of bowel habits invigorating. But a quick survey of the multitude of laxatives, bulking agents, stool softeners, and stimulants filling drugstore shelves is a dead giveaway—it's not just Grandma who's preoccupied with poop. Americans spend $725 million a year on laxatives alone. It seems we are all in search of the perfect bowel movement—some of us simply *a* bowel movement. But what *is* the perfect bowel movement (or BM, for those of us who were taught to initialize questionable terms for the sake of modesty)? What kind of bowel habits would keep me healthy and happy and far from the digestive aids aisle—the kind that would make Grandma proud?

What's a Normal BM?

Yes, ladies and gentlemen, I'm about to describe a normal bowel movement, an undertaking not to be taken lightly. First, why do we poop? A bowel movement occurs when feces present in the rectum cause distention, which then leads to reflex contraction of the smooth muscles of the rectum and relaxation of the anal sphincter. About this same time the abdominal and diaphragm muscles contract and the stool is expelled. Ideally, the abdomen will be completely comfortable until the time to eliminate, and then a pain-free urge will be felt in the lower abdomen. There is no panicked rush to the bathroom—no problem with a brief delay while locating the proper facilities. The bowel movement itself is painless, accompanied by a sense of pleasant relief, and occurs after one light abdominal push (no severe or repeated straining). Maximum "downloading time" will be less than ninety seconds (for the entire time on the toilet, including cleanup). A feeling of complete evacuation is experienced, and any further urge to defecate disappears until sometime later when the rectum is filled again.

The consistency of the feces should be soft and usually unformed—but the passage may be tubular—sausage shaped—and still be normal. Often the stool will break apart in the toilet bowl, and sometimes parts of the evacuation will float. Keep in mind that, contrary to popular thought (people *do* think about it), "floating feces" is not an indication that you are eating sufficient fiber. Not too long ago there was commercial bread in the supermarkets that got its high fiber content from the pulp of trees. Sure, these fecal "boats" produced as a result of eating pulverized oak tree toast would float in the toilet—but they were definitely not normal.

The color of stool produced by someone eating a plant-based diet is light yellow to brown. However, various vegetables can impart distinct colors. For example, beets will turn the stool dark red. The American diet loaded with iron-laden meats imparts the more familiar darker brown color to the stool. Incidentally, in a healthful fruits-and-vegetables diet, it is perfectly normal to have a bowel movement containing undigested plant parts, such as corn kernels, peas, and blueberries.

Most people have bowel movements one to three times a day, usually in the morning. However, others will easily pass their soft stool as infrequently as every other day—and this is right for them. Most important is the consistency of the matter and the ease with which it is eliminated. When first starting the McDougall Diet the bowels may seem overactive, but they settle down to a more normal pattern in one to two weeks as the body begins to adjust to this new, more healthful way of eating.

So there you have it, the perfect bowel movement. An ideal to which we all aspire. Now let's look at the grim reality that most Americans live with day in and day out.

Bowel Movements Gone Bad

Following my depiction of the perfect bowel movement, Larry's puzzled expression announced to me that the quick, painless process I'd described was completely foreign to him. Unfortunately, for most people like Larry living in Western societies, bathroom experiences rarely go as smoothly as they should. I'm reminded of the time my own children inadvertently made this discovery. Many years ago while enjoying a peaceful dinner one summer evening, our ten-year-old daughter, Heather, asked, "Is there something wrong with Jodi?" Heather and Patrick, our nine-year-old son, had spent the previous night at the home of their best friends, Jodi and Mark. Heather continued, "When Jodi's in the bathroom I hear these strange noises, like she's in horrible pain." She demonstrated with a long, painful grunting sound. Patrick interjected, "Mark makes the same noises, and he's in there forever." Our kids (who were born into the McDougall way of eating) found this strange.

For them this daily process was accomplished effortlessly and in seconds—back out to play before the ball stopped bouncing.

In societies where a Westernized diet is the norm, the urge to defecate can be accompanied by feelings ranging from mild discomfort to distressing pain in the mid to lower abdomen, while the bowel movement itself often requires prolonged muscular straining and can cause rectal pain and even bleeding. No wonder they call the toilet the "reading room." Larry boasted that he could finish two, sometimes three, Reader's Digest stories in the time it took to carry out the business at hand.

Constipation:
The All-American Movement

One of the most common bowel problems in American society is constipation, a condition characterized by difficult or infrequent passage of feces, hardness of stool, and/or a feeling of incomplete evacuation—*I think I'm finished . . . or am I?* Larry, like many others, couldn't remember a time in his life when he had been able to go to the bathroom without much straining and effort. Between 16 and 34 percent of children and 20 percent of people over the age of sixty-five reportedly suffer from chronic constipation. In addition, most people suffering from irritable bowel syndrome (IBS), which we will discuss later, report constipation as their primary symptom.

Dairy Binds the Bowels—Big Time

Once these less common, but medically significant, causes of constipation are ruled out, your primary attention should be focused on the connection between diet and constipation. Seems like a logical place to start, but somehow virtually the entire medical profession has missed the obvious—what you put in your intestines affects how they function. One of my medical textbooks states that constipation is caused by a failure to answer the urge to

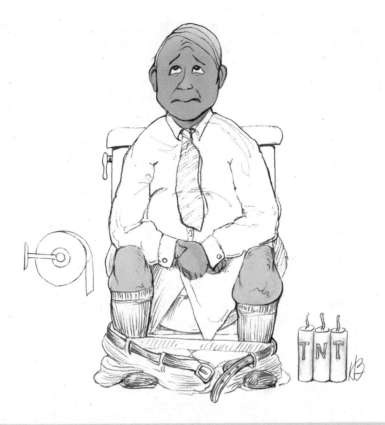

Dairy products will bind your bowels. No-fiber foods—beef, chicken, and fish make constipation a painful way of life. You are less than twenty-four hours away from relief with the McDougall Diet.

difficult, I challenge anyone to ignore the urge after following my dietary recommendations for just a couple of days.

Dairy protein can cause severe constipation. A 1998 study published in the *New England Journal of Medicine* looked at sixty-five severely constipated children averaging only one bowel movement every three to fifteen days. Though these children did not respond to strong laxatives (lactulose and mineral oil), forty-four of the sixty-five (68 percent) found relief of their constipation by removing cow's milk from their diet. Related problems, such as

Uncommon Causes of Constipation

First we will look at some important, but uncommon, causes of constipation that must be ruled out. The presence of some of these conditions should be brought to the attention of your doctor.

Anal fissures and hemorrhoids: These are painful conditions that can produce a spasm of the anal sphincter muscle. Subsequent fear of defecation then causes retained stool.

Systemic diseases: Constipation can result from diseases of the nervous tissues and muscles, such as scleroderma, multiple sclerosis, Parkinson's disease, spinal cord injuries, and stroke. Scarring, inflammation from diverticulitis, tumors, and cancer can produce mechanical compression of the intestine and sometimes complete bowel obstruction, thereby causing constipation. Metabolic disorders, such as dehydration, diabetes, and hypothyroidism, can also cause constipation.

Immobility and inconvenience: Injury or illness (especially when a bedpan is required) or a schedule that makes elimination inconvenient or unsociable will result in retained feces that become dehydrated and hard to pass.

Laxative use: Because of real or imagined constipation, many people become dependent upon laxatives. Stimulant laxatives are particularly troublesome because the bowel becomes dependent on this "artificial" stimulation and will not contract sufficiently with the normal reflexes caused by filling the rectum with stool.

Medications: Many medications, including pain medications (narcotics), antacids containing aluminum or calcium, antispasmodic drugs, antidepressant drugs, tranquilizers, iron supplements, anticonvulsants for epilepsy, antiparkinsonism drugs, and antihypertensive drugs (especially calcium channel blockers), commonly cause constipation.

Travel: Constipation due to travel is caused by changes in diet, water intake, and schedule. Conscious avoidance of unhealthful foods and constant rehydration alleviates this disturbance.

Pregnancy: Although pregnancy is a normal, healthy stage in a woman's life, many women become constipated as a result of the diet they are encouraged to adopt during pregnancy. Expectant mothers are often instructed to drink at least four glasses of milk a day and eat plenty of protein in the form of meat. You are about to learn why this is a prescription for constipation.

inflammation of the bowel, anal fissures, and pain, were all resolved as well with the elimination of cow's milk. When cow's milk was reintroduced into their diet eight to twelve months later, all of the children redeveloped constipation within five to ten days.

As a result of this allergic-type reaction to the protein in cow's milk, a child's bowels become paralyzed. Abdominal cramping and bloating become a routine part of the child's life. Because of the intense, continuous straining and rock-hard consistency of the bowel movement, the child often bleeds bright red blood into the toilet bowl and onto the toilet paper. The parents worry that something is not right, while the child, who *knows* something is not right, becomes embarrassed and ashamed that his or her bowel habits have become the focus of attention. Given the clear link between cow's milk and constipation, and in light of the distressing effects of constipation on children, government subsidized and sanctioned milk programs should be discontinued from schools nationwide.

The Fiber Factor

any people have the mistaken notion that fiber is like the abrasive bristles of a broom sweeping the intestines clean. Actually, dietary fiber is made of microscopic chains of sugar (carbohydrate) that pass all the way through the small intestine undigested, forming the bulk of the stool. The fiber pulls in water to further expand the volume of the stool, which contributes to large, soft, regular, pain-free bowel movements. Fiber also slows the absorption of calories and other nutrients through the bowel and into the body. This helps keep the body's blood sugar levels from becoming erratic and elevated and may play a role in controlling diabetes. Dietary fibers also bind and deactivate cancer-causing substances (such as environmental chemicals), as well as remove excess cholesterol and hormones. In an upcoming chapter you will learn how dietary fiber also helps your digestive system maintain a healthy level of "good" bacteria.

When there is little dietary fiber in your diet, there is little substance to form a stool (a few dead cells and a paltry amount of fiber). It is not surprising then that nearly 70 percent of adherents to the Atkins diet, which emphasizes high meat and dairy consumption with little dietary fiber, report constipation. The result is usually a few tiny, rock-hard fecal marbles eliminated biweekly. Not a pleasant bathroom scenario. Because these marbles are small in volume, they provide little distention of the rectum and are hard to evacuate—encouraging constipation.

Fiber is found only in plant foods. There is not a speck of fiber in beef, chicken, fish, lobster, eggs, milk, or cheese. On the conventional American diet, the few grains people do consume, like rice and flours, are highly refined into white rice and white flours that have lost most of their fiber content in the manufacturing process. The typical Western diet consists of 8–14 grams of dietary fiber a day. By contrast, the McDougall Diet provides 40–100 grams of daily dietary fiber.

Beyond the Fiber

At one point, Larry had actually tried sprinkling wheat bran on his breakfast—French toast with butter, fried hash browns, and even bacon, if you can believe it. A noble effort, but of course you can't just add fiber to an otherwise unhealthful diet and expect any kind of positive result. Besides, why ruin the taste of a perfectly greasy slab of bacon for no reason?

In order to have consistently normal bowel movements, you need to put the right things into your colon, which means putting the right foods on your table. A diet based on unrefined starches—like potatoes, beans, rice, corn, sweet potatoes, and whole wheat breads and pastas—with the addition of fruits and vegetables, is just what your digestive system needs to function properly. Animal products, especially dairy protein of any kind, will disrupt good bowel habits almost immediately, with normal function not returning until three to four days after discontinuing these foods and reintroducing healthful ones. Exercise and drinking more water have been suggested for relief of constipation, but their benefits are questionable.

Priming the Pump

Years of poor bowel function characterized by constipation can cause residual problems, such as bowel distention and a "lazy bowel," especially if there has also been laxative abuse. The bowel muscles are so weak they are no longer able to contract effectively. To make things worse, after years of being stimulated by the chemicals in laxatives, the bowel becomes insensitive to natural stimuli offered by the presence of stool and contracts only in the presence of this artificial stimulation.

How do you break the laxative habit and cure a "lazy bowel"? It takes some planning, patience, and, above all, training. The bowel must be brought back to its normal condition of contracting from the stimulus of fecal distention. It needs to be exercised so the muscles can grow strong again. The first step is to eat *plenty* of the right foods (this is no time for dieting). Fill the bowel with fiber and remove all paralyzing dairy proteins. It may take several days before the urgency to have a bowel movement hits. Be patient.

If after making the changes I have suggested you do not have a voluminous, soft movement within a week, or if you are suffering

Extra Help for Stubborn Bowels

Wheat bran can add bulk to the stool and encourage effortless bowel movements. This product can be purchased as "Miller's bran" or in various cereals advertised as "bran." *Fruits* add both dietary fiber and water to the diet. Some fruits, like prunes and kiwifruit, have mild stimulatory effects on the bowel, promoting bowel movements.

Fiber supplements, such as partially hydrolyzed guar gum (PHGG; SunFiber is one example) and wheat bran, produce improvements in IBS symptoms (abdominal pain and bowel habits). PHGG is better tolerated and preferred by patients over other kinds of fiber supplements.

Flaxseeds increase bowel movements by about 30 percent and can be consumed as a cereal (for example, Uncle Sam Cereal) or added to any grain before cooking (add 2–4 tablespoons of whole flaxseeds to each cup of grain). Flaxseeds may also reduce the risk for colon cancer.

Stool bulking agents increase the volume of the stool and can be used when more natural remedies (such as those listed above) are unsuccessful. You can buy these preparations without prescription: Metamucil, psyllium (ispaghula, isapgol, seed husks), methylcellulose (Citrucel), and sterculia.

Laxatives should be used only in moderation when absolutely necessary and usually under the direction of a physician. Bulking agents and osmotics (see below) are much preferred over stimulants because the bowel easily becomes dependent upon stimulants.

Stimulants, like castor oil, senna, dioctyl sodium sulfosuccinate (Dioctyl), Bisacodyl (Carter's Little Pills, Dulcolax, Fleet Bisacodyl), should be avoided. They eventually create laxative dependency.

Osmotic agents, such as lactulose, magnesium hydroxide, and magnesium sulfate, are an effective way to distend the bowel and safely stimulate movement when all else has been tried and failed. These should be used with a doctor's supervision.

Rectal enemas and suppositories, for example Dulcolax, glycerol suppositories, and phosphate enemas, should be used only for special needs under a doctor's supervision.

with abdominal pains or noticeable bleeding, then you should consult your doctor immediately. In addition, if you suspect at any time that something more than just lazy gut muscles are delaying normal function, then you should see your doctor—occasionally an obstruction from a tumor or a fecal impaction needs medical attention.

Sometimes it is necessary to "prime the pump" by artificially and purposefully overfilling the bowel. This can be done with wheat bran, psyllium seeds, flaxseeds, or as a last resort, with a nonabsorbable sugar called lactulose (doctor's prescription required). Ease and regularity of bowel movements should improve in the following days until movements are effortless, at which time the dosage of wheat bran, psyllium seeds, flaxseeds, and/or lactulose can be slowly decreased and eventually discontinued.

Larry Says Good-Bye to Laxatives

Louise joked that Larry had single-handedly kept the laxative manufacturers in business. "I'm looking forward to cleaning out the medicine cabinet to make room for necessities—like my beauty cream," she said.

Larry added, "I look forward to spending less time in the bathroom. Although I'm afraid I'll get a little behind in my reading once I'm consistently achieving 'the perfect bowel movement.'"

SUMMARY SHEET *from Dr. McDougall*

- *People on the Western diet commonly complain of difficult or infrequent passage of feces, hard stool, or a feeling of incomplete evacuation.*
- *The perfect BM is soft, unformed, light brown, and easy to pass.*
- *Frequency of movements can be from three times a day to every other day.*
- *There are several medical conditions that may cause constipation, and these may need to be discussed with your doctor.*
- *Dairy protein is a common cause of severe constipation—and this means low-fat milk, too.*
- *Dietary fiber, made of microscopic chains of sugar, provides ideal bulk for the bowels.*
- *Dietary fiber is only found in plant foods—never in beef, chicken, fish, shellfish, eggs, milk, or cheese.*
- *Refining grains to make white rice and flour removes nutritious dietary fiber.*
- *Dietary fiber speeds transition of the food and slows absorption of calories, aiding weight loss and helping to prevent diabetes.*
- *Dietary fibers deactivate cancer-causing substances and help remove excess cholesterol and hormones from the body.*
- *Lazy bowels, from years of constipation and laxatives, may take some extra effort, like added fiber (wheat bran, psyllium seeds, and/or flaxseeds) or lactulose, to fix.*
- *There are multiple agents that can be added to your bowel recovery program from bran to laxatives.*
- *If constipation is not easily resolved with a good diet, then see your doctor.*

CHAPTER 9

Bowel Sickness and the Fiber Factor

A s a senior medical student in the autumn of 1971, I sat in on a usual noontime hospital conference that would turn out to be a life-changing experience for me. I remember only one slide shown by visiting lecturer Dr. Denis Burkitt, the physician who discovered the immune system cancer named after him—Burkitt's Lymphoma. On one side of the slide was pictured a large hospital building with a small bowel movement next to it. In the adjacent frame was a small hospital beside a large bowel movement. He said, "America is a constipated nation . . . If you pass small stools, you have to have large hospitals." And according to Dr. Burkitt, the key to big bowel movements is a diet high in fiber. This was the *first* doctor who ever told me that diet and health were directly related—that the foods we consume can and do cause the majority of our most common chronic diseases.

Denis Burkitt, known as "The Fiber Man," set out in the mid-sixties to tell the world how important it was to eat a high-fiber diet. In fact, when I met Dr. Burkitt he was visiting the Kellogg Company in Battle Creek, Michigan, to try to convince them to add more dietary fiber to their cereal products. Dr. Burkitt's conclusions about the importance of dietary fiber were a result of observations made during his eighteen years as Government Surgeon of Uganda.

Dr. Burkitt observed that the African people produce several times more quantity of feces than people on the highly refined, meat-filled Western diet. He noticed their feces were soft and passed

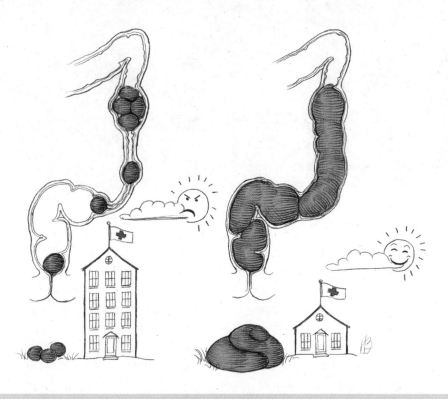

Reduce health-care costs and resolve diseases affecting hundreds of millions of people simply by making small bowel movements large.

without pain, and attributed this to the high fiber content of their foods. While Westerners have three to twenty-one bowel movements a week, passing 85–150 grams of feces per day (3–5 ounces), Africans have thirty to sixty movements a week, with a stool weight of 200–500 grams a day (7–17 ounces).

Most importantly, he noticed that the diseases he had been trained to treat in Scotland were absent among Africans. He saw no cases of type 2 diabetes, obesity, appendicitis, diverticular disease, hemorrhoids, dental caries, varicose veins, pulmonary embolism, inflammatory bowel diseases (Crohn's disease and ulcerative colitis), or hiatus hernia, and only one case of gallstones, in twenty years. He mused that the only incidence of heart attack he saw in nearly two decades was in a judge who had recently returned from his law school training in London, where he had developed a love for beef and other rich foods.

Eating a high-fiber diet is crucial to a healthy digestive system. But fiber alone cannot do the job. Though Dr. Burkitt was entirely correct about the role of fiber in maintaining digestive health, there are many other important qualities of the Africans' plant-based diet that contributed to their low incidence of chronic illness, such as their low fat intake. Dr. Burkitt himself often said, "The frying pan you should give to your enemy. Food should not be prepared in fat. Our bodies are adapted to a Stone Age diet of roots and vegetables."

The African diet has traditionally been a diet based on grains, legumes, vegetables, and fruits, with very little meat, dairy products, or refined foods. This means a diet very low in animal protein, fat, and cholesterol, and high in complex carbohydrates, dietary fiber, and healthful phytochemicals. These are the components of a healthful human diet, and by no coincidence, the foundation of the McDougall Diet.

Many "mysterious" diseases that plague people living on the Western diet are easily understood when you realize the importance of the foods you consume. This same understanding will lead you to prevent, and quite often to reverse, these conditions by making the right choices about what you put in your mouth. Here are some examples of common diseases that are the direct results of dietary choices.

Appendicitis

The contents of the small intestine empty into the large intestine. At about this junction a small pouch, or diverticulum called the appendix, is attached to the large intestine. When the opening of the appendix becomes irritated and blocked by unhealthful remnants of partially digested foods, fluids accumulate. These stagnant fluids become infected, creating a disease condition common to Westerners called appendicitis. Although appendicitis was once unknown among cultures such as those observed by Dr. Burkitt, whose diets were centered around plant foods, the incidence of this illness is increasing as these cultures adopt a more Westernized diet.

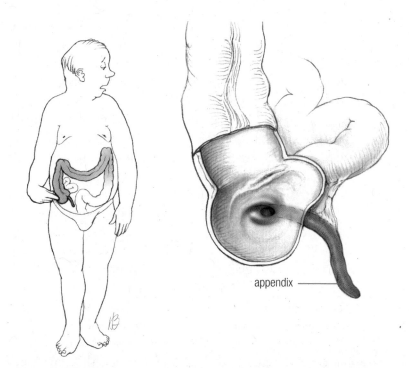

appendix ————

Appendicitis happens only to people who eat low-fiber foods. This pain in your right side can lead to an afternoon in the operating room.

Diverticular Disease

enis Burkitt, practicing in Uganda, and doctors taking care of populations of people following similar diets, never see diverticular disease. As food moves through the small intestine, the nutrients (protein, fats, carbohydrates, vitamins, and minerals) are absorbed through the intestinal wall into the bloodstream. Left behind are nondigestible matter (dietary fiber), colon bacteria, and many dead cells that will soon become the stool. This material passes into the right side of the large intestine and is then moved to the left side by rhythmic contractions known as peristalsis. According to the well-known law of physics, the Law of Laplace, contractions at small diameters cause high pressures. If there is minimal fiber in the diet, and therefore very little

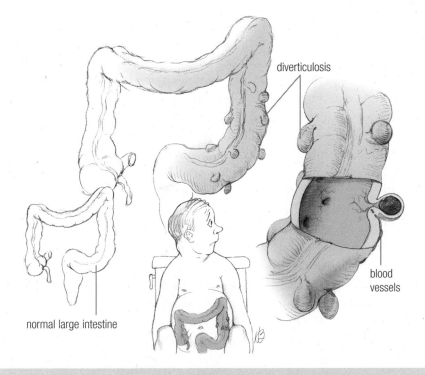

diverticulosis

blood vessels

normal large intestine

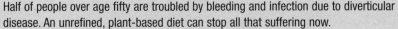

Half of people over age fifty are troubled by bleeding and infection due to diverticular disease. An unrefined, plant-based diet can stop all that suffering now.

stool mass, these contractions occur at high pressures. Years of elevated pressures produce ruptures in the walls of the intestine (balloon-like bulges) called *diverticula*. Half of people who have followed the Western diet for more than fifty years have diverticular disease.

The weaker parts of the intestinal wall are the areas where small blood vessels pass (or "dive") from the outer surface through the muscular wall and into the inner surface of the intestine. These areas of weakness are the most common locations for diverticula to develop. Because of the proximity of the diverticula to blood vessels in the intestine, one of the primary symptoms of this disease is bleeding (blood is found in the stool because there is bleeding into the gut). I have seen the bleeding so severe that the only way to save the patient's life was to surgically remove a sizeable portion of the large intestine.

When the diverticula become irritated by the unhealthful remnants of digested food, the openings in them can close up, allowing the fluids to become stagnant and infected—a condition known as *diverticulitis*. This disease is sometimes referred to as "left-sided appendicitis" (remember the real appendix is located in the right lower part of the abdomen), and is usually treated with antibiotics. Switching to a high-fiber diet will greatly reduce the risk of future bleeding and infection; however, the diverticula do not disappear with a change in diet. The commonly held notion that nuts and seeds get caught in diverticula and cause diverticulitis is unsupported by any scientific research and is untrue.

Larry informed me that he had been diagnosed with diverticulosis four years earlier and had been on several rounds of antibiotics in an effort to control his symptoms. (Diverticulosis is the condition without infection. It involves just the pouches, though they still may bleed. Diverticulitis is the condition when the pouches are infected.) I assured him that he would likely find the relief he'd been seeking for so long by switching to the plant-based, high-fiber diet Louise had resolved to follow.

Hemorrhoids

Picture a person seated on the toilet grunting and groaning, face bright red. The face isn't the only recipient of a high-pressure blood rush. A ring of internal veins around the anus, the hemorrhoidal veins, provides a compressible lining that allows the anus to completely close, a function that, let's just say, helps us avoid some socially embarrassing situations involving flatulence and loss of bowel control. Hemorrhoids develop when straining to pass small, hard stools causes high retrograde pressures into these hemorrhoidal veins, causing them to dilate.

Eventually, after years of straining, these veins are permanently enlarged and commonly hang out the end of the anus. Sorry . . . can you think of a more delicate way to say it? This is where Larry found himself . . . with constant itching and burning, not to mention the bleeding that occurred with almost every bowel movement. "Dr. McDougall, I want to go to the bathroom, but I dread it too. I know it's going to hurt every time; I just never know how much or if it's going to bleed."

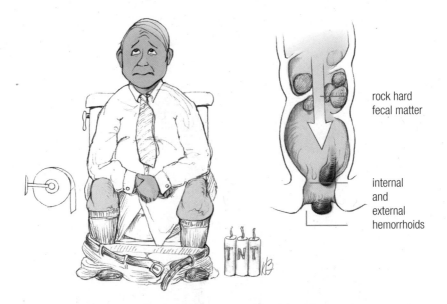

rock hard
fecal matter

internal
and
external
hemorrhoids

This pain in the rear is caused by straining to pass a constipated stool. Don't blame hemorrhoids from sitting on cold chairs. The itching and pain can be relieved by changing your diet.

"Larry," I told him, "you don't have to suffer like this. With a change in diet, you can probably relieve your current pain and avoid the later stages of hemorrhoid development, including the displacement of the anal muscles toward the outside." That was a scenario he definitely did not wish to see played out.

Although hemorrhoids are permanent structural changes, a surgical procedure called a hemorrhoidectomy can counter this damage through removal of some of the stretched-out tissue. Other procedures for troublesome hemorrhoids include sclerotherapy (injection with a caustic substance), photocoagulation, rubber band ligation, cryotherapy (freezing), and cutting with a laser. (Laser surgery is no less painful than traditional surgery and is more expensive.)

Hemorrhoid sufferers can often avoid invasive surgery and find relief from their symptoms (pain, itching, and bleeding) through the use of topical cleansers and creams, sitting in warm baths (sitz baths), and most importantly through making better food choices.

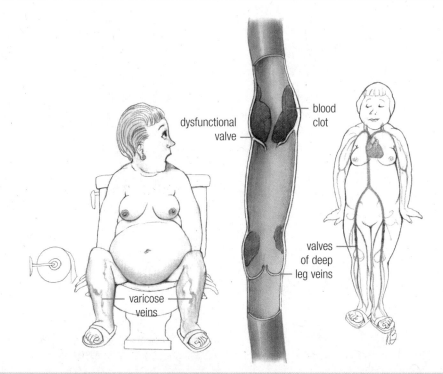

These dilated "blue worms" crawling over your legs should not be blamed on pregnancy or standing. Varicose veins are from destructive forces caused by years of difficult bowel movements.

Interestingly, hemorrhoids used to be a rare occurrence in rural Africa. But as Africans have switched to a modern diet, approximately one-fifth now have these dilated veins.

Varicose Veins

Notice that when you are standing, the distance from your feet to your heart is about four to five feet. A column of blood this tall would place tremendous pressure on the veins of the lower legs and feet if not for special valves that shut closed to prevent flow of the blood in the direction of the feet. The muscles in the legs contract when we walk, pushing blood upward and past the open valves toward the heart. These valves carry blood only one way, and

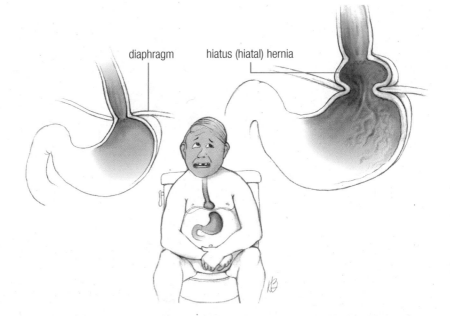

Suffering with a hiatus (hiatal) hernia is so common that people think it comes with age. Many years of straining on the toilet eventually push the stomach up into the chest.

as they close, they prevent blood from falling back down toward the feet. As many as three-fourths of women and half of men following the Western diet have varicose veins. Not surprisingly, people who have varicose veins are more likely to suffer from hemorrhoids—the conditions have the same dietary cause.

Hiatus (Hiatal) Hernia

The act of having a bowel movement raises the pressures in the abdominal cavity much higher than the pressures that are in the chest, pushing the stomach up into the chest cavity, creating a *hiatus (hiatal) hernia*. Half of people who have followed the Western diet for more than fifty years have some degree of hiatal hernia. The chest and the abdomen are separated anatomically by a large muscle used for breathing called the diaphragm. Three structures pass though the diaphragm—the aorta, vena cava, and esophagus.

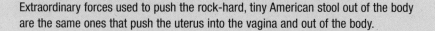

prolapsed
uterus

vaginal
wall

Extraordinary forces used to push the rock-hard, tiny American stool out of the body
are the same ones that push the uterus into the vagina and out of the body.

Only the esophagus is moveable. Straining pushes the stomach into
the natural opening for the esophagus, causing the muscular opening to dilate. A dilated muscle is known as a *hernia*. Eventually the
top portion of the stomach sits in the chest cavity, where each
breath creates negative pressures that draw acid up into the esophagus. With the stomach out of its natural position supported by the
diaphragm muscle, the lower esophageal sphincter (LES), which
functions to close the opening between the esophagus and stomach,
is rendered incompetent. (See Chapter 4, pages 25–26, to learn
more about LES dysfunction and resulting GERD.)

Surgical repair can move the stomach back into the abdominal
cavity and close the hernia. However, this operation should be
reserved for those who cannot find relief from a healthful diet, raising the head of their bed, and/or antacids.

Other Bowel-Related Conditions

Other conditions caused or aggravated by continued straining during bowel movements include prolapse of the female uterus, spermatocele (dilation of the spermatic cord), cystocele (prolapse of the female bladder), and rectocele (prolapse of the rectum).

Treatment of Damaged Tissues

Unfortunately, the structural changes caused by straining are permanent and will not return to normal with a change in diet. However, a healthful diet will relieve most of the uncomfortable symptoms and problems associated with diverticulosis (bleeding and infection), hemorrhoids (bleeding, pain, and itching), and hiatus hernia (heartburn). Surgery for these and other conditions discussed should be an option chosen only after trying less drastic measures for relief, most importantly a change in diet.

Take It Easy on Your Body

By the end of our "bowel visit," as the Bortons jokingly referred to it, Louise had reconfirmed her commitment to sticking with the McDougall Diet, stating that when she ate the foods I suggested she felt better—her bloating and abdominal cramps disappeared, and she'd had fun fitting into clothes she hadn't worn for years. "Most of all," she said, "I stopped having a dysfunctional love-hate relationship with the bathroom!"

Larry, on the other hand, was less enthusiastic. He wasn't motivated by the benefits of healthful eating since, unlike Louise, he hadn't adhered to my guidelines for more than a few days, and even then admitted to having had a stash of goodies (buttered popcorn, beef jerky, canned spray cheese, and crackers) at work. Before leaving my office, he did manage to scrape up a halfhearted, "Yeah, I'll do the diet," and departed with these words, "Doc, are you sure there's no fiber in donuts?"

SUMMARY SHEET *from Dr. McDougall*

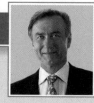

- Denis Burkitt, the "Fiber Man," changed my professional life—he opened my eyes to the dietary cause of common diseases.

- Only plant foods contain dietary fiber.

- Straining to pass a tiny, rock-hard stool damages tissues from head to toe.

- Appendicitis is due to infection, secondary to blockage caused by irritating forces from foods on the Western diet.

- Diverticulosis is due to high internal bowel pressures from tiny stools resulting from a diet pitifully deficient in undigestible carbohydrates (dietary fiber).

- Hemorrhoids are veins distended by years of forceful straining on the toilet.

- Varicose veins form when the valves within the leg veins are damaged through years of straining to move the bowels.

- A hiatus hernia results from the stomach being forced upward by efforts to move a stubborn stool downward.

- The lower esophageal sphincter (LES) becomes incompetent when it is displaced and no longer supported by the muscular diaphragm.

- GERD (acid reflux) occurs when the LES becomes incompetent.

- Other disorders from years of straining include prolapse of the female uterus, spermatocele (dilation of the spermatic cord), cystocele (prolapse of the female bladder), and rectocele (prolapse of the rectum).

- A healthful diet will provide considerable relief from the disorders caused by constipation, and this simple approach should be tried first.

- Since these are structural changes (damage), mechanical methods, like surgery, may be required as the last resort for relief.

CHAPTER 10

Chained to the Bathroom with Colitis

At the opposite end of the spectrum from our previous discussion on constipation is the scenario depicted in the popular TV ad for antidiarrheal medication—a desperate, panic-stricken guy on the street frantically searching for a public restroom accompanied by the catchy tune, "Gotta go, gotta go, gotta go right now!" Who can't recall the sudden, painful assault of "traveler's diarrhea," or the paralyzing fear of a public display of fecal matter with a bad case of stomach flu? Can you imagine this happening almost every day—all day long?

Unfortunately, for people like Louise, this is a way of life. Abdominal cramping, along with unannounced bouts of diarrhea (sometimes with blood and mucus) was the reason for Louise's appointment that day. After addressing her concerns about Larry's bowel problems, and learning more about constipation than they'd ever dreamed of knowing, we were ready to turn to Louise's pressing health issue.

"Dr. McDougall, I am that person in the commercial trying to find a bathroom before the unthinkable occurs. Actually, there have been a couple of times I didn't quite make it. It's humiliating and horrifying. I never know when it's going to hit, unless it's one of those times when I'm doubled over in pain beforehand."

Louise's usual sense of humor gave way to genuine concern and discouragement. Tears formed in her eyes as she shared with me how this illness had robbed her of the ability to enjoy her life.

"I love teaching, Dr. McDougall. But I find myself watching the clock at school now, counting the minutes until I can get home where I won't have to worry about whether there's a toilet nearby. My daughter and I haven't met for our regular girls' night out for weeks. I should have called you sooner, but I kept thinking I just had a virus that would go away. It's not going away. I'm scared, Dr. McDougall."

I've heard countless stories just like Louise's throughout my years of medical practice. Each time my heart breaks for these fine people whose lives are hijacked by this painful illness that inflicts such shame and suffering.

"Louise, the important thing is you're here now, and that's the first step toward getting better. What you're describing is an illness called colitis, an inflammation of the large intestine. Colitis can be caused by a bacterial infection, parasites, a virus, medications, or even an allergic reaction to food and other substances we ingest."

As I explained to Louise, the offending agent that causes colitis can enter the colon from the remnants of food flowing inside the intestine or through the bloodstream. When the colitis is short-lived, there is usually full recovery with no serious consequences. However, there are chronic forms of colitis that never go away and are resistant to all the drugs modern medicine has to offer. Chronic colitis can range from very mild and hardly noticeable to severe and life-threatening, with all levels in between.

Mild chronic colitis is most often referred to as irritable bowel syndrome (IBS), but is also known as spastic colitis and spastic colon. This disorder accounts for nearly 50 percent of referrals to gastroenterologists. IBS affects mostly women and is seen in as many as 24 percent of women and 15 percent of men in Western societies.

The primary symptoms of IBS are abdominal pain, bloating, feeling of incomplete evacuation, and poor bowel function. This may present with either diarrhea, as in Louise's case, or constipation as the predominant factor, or alternation between these two extremes. IBS sufferers find themselves chained to the bathroom either way—with random bouts of diarrhea or with prolonged efforts at producing some manner of bowel movement.

Drug Therapy for IBS Is a Killer

Louise was sure she'd found the simple solution to her IBS. "Dr. McDougall, the other day I saw Kelsey Grammer, the guy that used to be on the sitcom Frasier, with his wife on the *Today Show* talking about IBS; and I have seen lots of advertisements about this wonder drug for IBS called Lotronex. Frasier was a psychiatrist, a medical doctor, on TV, you know, so he wouldn't steer me wrong. If you'll just write me out a prescription, my bowel troubles will be over."

I hated to burst her bubble. "Louise, Kelsey Grammer had a little incentive to say good things about that drug. He was part of a celebrity campaign sponsored by the company that makes Lotronex, the brand name for the generic alosetron. Using famous people is just one part of the industry's strategy to promote Lotronex—their plan also includes doctors, advertisements, medical education conferences, medical guidelines, patient groups, and even unethical influence on the FDA. And their efforts are paying off. Lotronex and similar 'blockbuster' drugs, like Zelnorm, are a $10 billion business."

"Yeah, I saw Lynda Carter, the Wonder Woman, advertising that one."

"Louise, it would be great if this were indeed the miracle drug it's purported to be, but the fact is there are lots of problems with these kinds of medications. Basically it all boils down to this—they are of very little benefit and have side effects like severe constipation, bowel perforation leading to infection inside the body, and bowel infarction, which is like a heart attack to the bowel. Women have died as a result of taking this type of drug.

"OK, OK, I'm convinced. No such thing as an IBS miracle drug. But, Dr. McDougall, I can't go on suffering like this. I hope you have an alternative."

You may relate to Louise's desire to find a quick fix—a miracle drug that will cure your ills with no further effort. As with most other ailments of the body, minor or serious, the most effective, long-term treatment is usually found on the dinner table.

Dietary Treatment of Mild Colitis

With specific food intolerances indicated in as much as 58 percent of IBS cases (the most likely offenders being milk, wheat, and eggs), it just makes sense to begin here on the journey back to a healthy colon. There are many characteristics of the typical Western diet that can trigger this mild inflammation. This rich diet is high in fat and indigestible milk sugar (lactose), and low in fiber, carbohydrates, and plant chemicals (phytochemicals).

As with constipation sufferers, patients suffering from IBS can find significant improvement of their symptoms simply by adding fiber to their diet. However, it should be noted that patients with "predominant constipation-type" IBS experience significantly more improvement with fiber supplements than those with "predominant diarrhea." While most experiments in this regard have involved supplements of wheat bran or guar gum, I have seen greater benefits from switching to a plant-based diet, which yields a wide variety of naturally healthful dietary fibers rather than one single fiber source.

IBS has also been effectively treated with the introduction of "friendly intestinal bacteria" called *probiotics*. In one study, all patients treated with the organism *Lactobacillus plantarum* reported full resolution of abdominal pain, while half reported relief of constipation. Bowel-friendly bacteria thrive in a bowel filled with the remnants of starches, vegetables, and fruits, because their preferred food is carbohydrate (dietary fiber). Almost all of my patients find immediate relief of bowel cramps, diarrhea, and constipation by simply changing to the McDougall Diet—and these benefits are seen in less than two weeks.

Could It Be Celiac Disease?

Intestinal problems that linger despite adherence to the McDougall Diet may be the result of celiac disease. About 10 percent of people with IBS (and as many as 1 percent of the entire population) will also have celiac disease, a condition caused

Health Problems More Common with Celiac Disease

AUTOIMMUNE DISEASES:

- Type 1 diabetes
- Hypothyroidism
- Hyperthyroidism
- Sjögren's syndrome
- Scleroderma
- Rheumatoid arthritis

- Psoriasis
- Lupus
- Alopecia (hair loss)
- Adrenal insufficiency
- Vasculitis

NON-AUTOIMMUNE DISEASES:

- Lymphomas
- Other cancers
- Dermatitis herpetiformis (severe dermatitis)
- Skin burning, prickling, itching, or tingling
- Bone loss (osteopenia)
- Loss of dental enamel
- Anemia (iron deficiency)
- Fetal loss

- Liver dysfunction (elevated enzymes)
- Growth retardation
- Infertility
- Delayed puberty
- Neurologic disorders (cerebellar ataxia, migraine, neuropathy, epilepsy)
- Autism
- Schizophrenia

by gluten—protein molecules most commonly found in wheat, barley, and rye. After sugar, gluten is the second most prevalent food substance in Western civilization. Celiac disease prevents the small intestine from effectively absorbing necessary nutrients. This malabsorption then leads to diarrhea, abdominal pain, flatulence, weakness, and weight loss. In late stages, nutritional deficiencies can result. There is a genetic tendency to develop celiac disease, but breastfeeding and the introduction of gluten after the first three months of life both reduce future risk.

Offending Foods for Celiac Disease

- Barley
- Kamut
- Rye
- Spelt
- Triticale
- Wheat (durum, semolina, bulgur, seitan*)
- Beer, ales, and malted drinks contain considerable gluten.

* The vegetarian meat substitute called seitan is made of gluten concentrate.

Lactobacilli bacteria, which are used to make sourdough bread, remove (hydrolyze) most of the gluten and make the wheat tolerable for most people with celiac disease.

The first step in confirming a clinical suspicion of celiac disease, based on the patient's story, is a blood test to measure levels of immunoglobulin A antibodies (IgA), anti-tissue transglutaminase (tTGA), or IgA antiendomysium antibodies (AEA). If the patient has been eating gluten regularly and all three tests come back positive, there is a very high chance that the patient has celiac disease. However, the diagnosis is only confirmed when a biopsy of the intestine shows classic changes characteristic of celiac disease. The connection between gluten and this disease is so clear that diagnosis can also be made if the patient experiences dramatic improvement of symptoms upon following a gluten-free diet.

People with untreated celiac disease have a two to six times greater risk of dying, mainly due to an increase in the risk of lymphoma. People with celiac disease also have a much greater risk of suffering from autoimmune diseases, like type 1 diabetes and thyroiditis. The reason for an increase in additional diseases probably lies with the damage to the intestine that allows the unfiltered passage of viruses, bacteria, and food proteins into the body.

Foods Acceptable for Celiac Disease

GRAINS:

- Amaranth
- Buckwheat (kasha)
- Corn
- Job's tears
- Millet
- Oats*

- Quinoa
- Rice
- Sorghum
- Teff
- Wild rice

* Oats have been demonstrated in multiple studies to be free of toxic proteins and tolerated by most (but not all) people with celiac disease, but there is worry that commercial oat products may be contaminated with wheat.

OTHER FOODS:

- Root vegetables, like potatoes, yams, sweet potatoes, and cassava root (tapioca)
- All legumes (beans, peas, and lentils)*
- All green and yellow vegetables
- All fruits

*Legumes make extra gas, sometimes causing bloating and bowel discomfort.

Diet: The Only Treatment for Celiac Disease

Celiac disease is a lifelong condition—therefore patients must stick to a diet low in gluten in order to regain and maintain lost health. As with all dietary treatments, lack of compliance, usually due to insufficient motivation and information, is the greatest obstacle to overcome.

Once diagnosed with celiac disease, many individuals attempt to replace familiar foods like breads and noodles with gluten-free varieties. Unfortunately, some of these same people complain that the gluten-free products are not as tasty as the originals. You might try "spaghetti" noodles made from rice, corn, quinoa, or buckwheat. Use corn tortillas instead of wheat flour wraps. Though it may take some time to find suitable gluten-free alternatives for favorite foods, the result is well worth the effort—simple, cost-free, side-effect-free relief from a serious, lifelong condition.

Why Is Chronic Colitis Incurable?

Severe forms of colitis are known as *inflammatory bowel disease* (IBD) and encompass two categories of disease called *ulcerative colitis* (UC) and *Crohn's disease* (CD). These diseases so closely resemble each other that it is often difficult for doctors to distinguish between them. IBD is an autoimmune disease in which the body attacks its own bowel tissues, causing symptoms of abdominal pain, bloody diarrhea, and mucus—sometimes leading to surgery and death. The diagnosis is made in part by a process of elimination when examinations, including cultures for bacteria and parasites, uncover no other cause.

This form of colitis is chronic because the source of the inflammation continues its attack, causing unrelenting injury to the colon. Obviously, the ultimate solution to this chronic condition would be to isolate the offending agent and eliminate it. Modern medicine can do this effectively with cases of parasite infections, such as giardia, by killing the parasites with the aid of antibiotics. But most cases of chronic colitis are incurable because the offending agent(s) remains elusive.

In practical terms, modern medicine fails patients with IBD for one primary reason—most practicing doctors refuse to consider the obvious connection between diet and these kinds of digestive ailments. IBD patients are told by their doctors, "Diet has nothing to do with this disease." Consider this—all doctors will readily admit that inhaling toxic elements from cigarettes damages the lungs, and drinking a quart of whiskey daily will destroy the liver. Yet somehow these learned authorities stubbornly deny that the digestive materials that remain for hours and sometimes days inside the intestinal tract could have any impact on this organ's health. How can such a logical connection be so blatantly disregarded?

IBD and Dietary Causes

Worldwide, IBD is more commonly found in northern than in southern populations, a trend that reflects patterns of consumption of the Western diet. In fact, IBD is found exclusively in societies where people consume a Westernized diet. Research shows that patients with IBD are more likely to consume meat, milk, fat, and refined food, and less likely to consume fruits and vegetables. Patients with UC are likely to have symptoms induced by cow's milk. A study involving UC patients in Japan found higher-fat diets were associated with two and a half times the risk of developing IBD—even so-called "good fats," like omega-3, olive oil, and other vegetable fats, increased the risk for developing these diseases. Thus, for prevention and treatment of IBD, your diet should be low in all kinds of fats.

Sulfur compounds may also play an important role in the cause of IBD. Hydrogen sulfide is toxic to the cells of the colon. This substance is produced in the bowel by the action of bacteria on dietary sources of sulfur—more specifically, sulfur-containing amino acids. Animal products are the main sources of these kinds of amino acids. If you'll recall our earlier discussion on bad breath—beef contains four times more sulfur than pinto beans, cheddar cheese contains five times more than white potatoes, and tuna contains twelve times more than sweet potatoes.

Contrary to prevailing medical "wisdom," evidence shows that diet is indeed the key causative factor of severe forms of colitis. Specifically, animal foods are the most harmful to the colon due to many factors, including high fat content, lack of fiber, allergic properties, and sulfur-containing amino acids.

Dietary Treatment of Severe Colitis

Very basic diets, called *elemental diets,* consisting of mostly sugar and water, have been found very effective in relieving acute flare-ups of Crohn's disease. This benefit is likely due to the absence of intact animal protein that would cause an autoimmune reaction with the gut. In one study comparing formulas with no intact protein with a formula containing intact milk protein, remission of symptoms occurred in only 36 percent of those taking the milk-protein formula, while 75 percent of those taking the protein-free formula enjoyed full resolution of their symptoms. Dietary fats have also been found to greatly reduce the benefits of an elemental diet.

One of the first thorough studies of patients with CD found two-thirds of patients treated with a healthful diet were well after two years. In one recent controlled study involving ninety-three CD patients, 84 percent achieved remission after two weeks of following an elimination diet. Predominant food intolerances discovered during this study were cereals, dairy products, and yeast.

Crohn's disease patients suffering from severe diarrhea (twenty or more stools per day) find relief from watery stools within two to three days when they are switched from a high-fat to a low-fat diet. Patients with CD have often suffered damage to the last part of their small intestine (ilium). As a result of this damage, bile from the liver that is normally reabsorbed by a *healthy* small intestine is instead allowed to pass directly into the large intestine. Here the bile acid causes severe irritation, with discharge of blood, mucus, and water. As long as thirty years ago, evidence showed that a low-fat diet can bring immediate relief to these patients, as bile acid production is decreased, thereby reducing irritation of the large intestine. In addition, the fiber introduced in a plant-based diet binds and neutralizes many of the bile acids and absorbs free water present in the stool.

Breaking the Chain to the Bathroom

Many early studies have shown that patients with UC and CD greatly benefit from a low-fat, plant-based diet. The best way to prevent and treat all forms of colitis, from mild to severe, is to eliminate all free fats (vegetable oils) and animal products, and to begin consuming a diet based on starches, with the addition of fruits and vegetables. In the unlikely event that these dietary considerations fail to cure colitis, the next step is to eliminate all wheat products.

Finally, the elimination diet (see page 104) should be employed in order to pinpoint any offending foods. Using this approach, I have seen most patients with colitis improve, many to the point of complete cure, including those with the more serious forms of IBD.

Louise Comes Clean

You might be asking yourself why Louise was in such distress when she had previously recommitted to eating healthful foods so she could keep her gallbladder. I had a hunch, but I was waiting to hear it from Louise. Before I could press the issue, Larry spoke up.

"Doc, she's already eating pretty much all the foods you told us to. What else is she supposed to do?"

Louise responded before I could answer. "Larry, you're right. I am eating the foods Dr. McDougall suggested—that's why I thought my symptoms were from some kind of virus that kept hanging on. The problem is I've also been eating some of the things he said not to. I really didn't think having milk on my cereal, or a little cheese on my salad, or coffee with half-and-half would make that big a difference. From what Dr. McDougall just told us, those dairy products, even in small amounts, are the very things causing me such misery."

"Louise," I explained, "dairy proteins often cause allergic-type reactions, and a little bit can do a lot of harm. Besides, you may think it's only a little here and there, but you eat salad quite often and you have coffee and cereal every day, maybe more than once, right?"

"Right, especially the coffee."

"So there is a steady stream of offensive food irritating your colon and disrupting your entire life. You just need to be introduced to some delicious, healthful alternatives so you won't feel the need to consume the bad stuff."

Louise took great comfort in knowing the reason for her distress and that she could do something about it. I set up a meeting between Louise and Mary, my wife and originator of most of the mouthwatering recipes in our program, so that Mary could personally suggest some specific alternatives to Louise's unhealthful choices.

A Highly Effective Elimination Diet (Foods Allowed)

COOKED STARCHES

- Brown rice
- Sweet potatoes
- Winter squash
- Taro (or poi)
- Tapioca flour
- Puffed rice

COOKED GREEN AND YELLOW VEGETABLES*

- Asparagus
- Artichokes
- Beets
- Beet greens
- Broccoli
- Chard
- Celery
- Kale
- Lettuce
- Spinach
- String beans
- Summer squash

*Avoid onions, green peppers, cucumbers, and radishes; they can be very troublesome for the stomach, causing indigestion.

COOKED FRUITS*

- Apples
- Apricots
- Bananas
- Cherries
- Cranberries
- Papaya
- Peaches
- Plums
- Prunes

*Avoid all citrus fruits (including oranges, grapefruits, tangerines, lemons, and limes) and tomatoes.

CONDIMENTS

Only salt is allowed (if not restricted for other health reasons). This means no salad dressings, mustard, lemon juice, vinegar, pepper, or other condiments.

BEVERAGES

Water (sparkling water is OK)

After one week with your digestive system free of offensive foods, you should be feeling well. If this is the case, you can begin adding other foods back to your diet—but be sure to *add only one new food item at a time*. This way, if you experience negative reactions, you will be able to pinpoint the specific food that should be avoided. For testing purposes, each new food should be eaten in large amounts three times a day for two days. If the food does not cause a reaction, you can conclude that it is not a troublemaker. Most reactions occur within a few hours, but some may not show up for several days. When you do have a reaction to a specific food, you must wait four to seven days before testing the next item. This interval gives your body ample time to rid itself of the effects of the allergy-causing food.

From years of experience dealing with wonderful people just like Louise, I knew that she would continue to make progress and soon learn enough from my advice to stay out of trouble. Eventually, my plan for her and for Larry (as with all my patients) is for them to become so accustomed to the fresh, unprocessed, healthful foods included in the McDougall Diet that they will never go back to their old ways of eating.

SUMMARY SHEET *from Dr. McDougall*

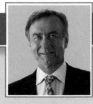

- *Colitis, inflammation of the colon, can be mild to severe and is caused by the contents of the colon.*

- *Mild chronic colitis is most often referred to as irritable bowel syndrome (IBS), and is also known as spastic colitis and spastic colon.*

- *Dairy products are among the most offending foods causing IBS.*

- *IBS is effectively treated with a healthful plant-based diet and sometimes probiotics.*

- *Celiac disease is caused by wheat, barley, and rye and is easily cured.*

- *Lymphomas and autoimmune diseases (type 1 diabetes and thyroiditis) are commonly associated with celiac disease.*

- *Severe forms of colitis are known as inflammatory bowel disease (IBD) and encompass two categories called ulcerative colitis (UC) and Crohn's disease (CD).*

- *IBD is found exclusively in people following the Western diet.*

- *Animal products are the most offensive components of the Western diet for many reasons—high fat, high protein, lack of fiber, allergic qualities, sulfur content, infectious agents, influence on bowel bacteria, and more.*

- *A person suffering from severe diarrhea (twenty or more stools per day) due to CD can find relief in two to three days by consuming a low-fat diet.*

- *Though rarely recommended by medical professionals, dietary change is a scientifically established effective treatment for IBD.*

- *The elimination diet is a highly effective last-step treatment for IBD—cost-free, side-effect-free, and patient-controlled.*

CHAPTER 11

Colon Polyps and Cancer

THE GUT SAYS, "ENOUGH!"

After learning that even a little forbidden food can wreak a lot of havoc on the digestive system, Louise was able to make those last adjustments in her dietary habits and find relief from her colitis. Unfortunately, her newfound commitment to healthful eating was not contagious. Larry continued his love affair with fried foods, one of his favorites being chicken-fried steak, which he was forced to obtain from a local restaurant since Louise was waging an all-out assault on fatty foods. In fairness to Larry, he did switch from chocolate-covered doughnuts to bran muffins on occasion, a well-intentioned but marginally effective adjustment. Larry finally got serious about a different way of eating when he sat in my office describing his latest symptoms.

"Dr. McDougall, it seems like my gut always aches—so bad that all I can do sometimes is curl up on the couch." I knew that feeling only too well. His brow furrowed as he continued. "But last week . . . I noticed . . . well, there was blood when I went to the bathroom. I don't mean a little bit, like when my diverticulosis acts up or my hemorrhoids. I'm talking about a lot of blood. There's never been this much before. Between the stabbing pain and the blood, I'm afraid something serious is wrong, Dr. McDougall."

Years of dietary abuse to his digestive system had led to this point—Larry would have to undergo tests to determine if he was suffering from colon polyps or worse—cancer of the colon.

107

In the Western world, colon cancer (also known as colorectal cancer) is the second most common form of deadly cancer. Each year in the United States and Europe 130,000 to 180,000 new cases are diagnosed. A person over fifty years of age has about a 5 percent chance over the remainder of his or her lifetime of developing colon cancer, and a 2.5 percent chance of dying of the disease. Unfortunately, due to the ineffectiveness of the most modern treatments, only about 40 percent of those diagnosed are still alive after five years.

Colon cancer arises from polyps (also called adenomas). In autopsy studies, approximately 35 percent of people consuming the typical Western diet are found to have colon polyps. Whether in the intestine, sinus cavities, or female cervix, polyps are distinct growths of excess tissue resulting from cellular proliferation of mucous membranes. They occur in response to constant irritation—in the same way calluses develop on the hands in an attempt to protect themselves from irritation.

By now you've probably learned enough about the digestive system to know the source of this irritation. The remnants of partially digested unhealthful foods that sit in the intestine are the starting point for these polyps. The size of the polyp when discovered is an indication of the strength and duration of the irritation.

The progression through which serious disease develops is as follows: irritation, cell proliferation, polyp development, and finally cancer. Large polyps, which are further along this developmental sequence, are more likely to be cancerous. Polyps less than 5 mm (one-half inch) are not likely to be cancerous, while 1 percent of polyps 10 mm in size show cancerous changes, increasing to 17 percent at 20 mm.

The key to preventing polyp formation, slowing their growth, preventing their transition to cancer, and possibly slowing the growth of the cancer even after it is started, is to stop the irritation of the mucosa of the intestine. In other words, your goal is to bathe the walls of your intestine with friendly foodstuffs, as soft and gentle as fluffy mashed potatoes.

Transition time from the earliest changes in the mucous membranes to the beginning of actual cancer takes, on average, ten to fifteen years. Less than one in twenty small polyps will grow larger and transform into cancer. Once the cancer begins, the time for metastasis (spreading to other parts of the body) and finally death takes another ten to twenty years. Therefore, the whole process from normal cells to cancer and death, if treatment is ineffective, will span, on average, twenty to thirty-five years. This is one reason colon cancer is primarily a disease of older people.

Who Gets Colon Cancer?

About 75 percent of people diagnosed with colon cancer have no predisposing characteristics other than their diet. The other 25 percent have conditions such as inflammatory bowel disease or a family history of colon cancer that puts them at higher-than-average risk. People with one or two first-degree relatives (parents, brothers, sisters) with colon cancer have twice the general risk of developing this disease. The question that remains unanswered is this: Does heredity pass on the predisposition for colon cancer through genetics, or is the strong familial pattern of common dietary habits (i.e., parents teach sons and daughters how to cook and what foods to enjoy) the culprit?

Food Is What's Eating You

Looking for evidence of the cause-effect relationship between diet and cancer, researchers uncovered a fifty-fold variation in the incidence of colon cancer worldwide. In countries where people eat rich diets—lots of meat, dairy, fats, sugars, and processed foods—there were high rates of polyps and colon cancer. Conversely a high intake of starches, fruits, and vegetables was associated with a low risk of these colon problems.

Our friend "The Fiber Man," Dr. Denis Burkitt, saw this diet/cancer connection firsthand during his work in Africa. Dr. Burkitt observed that African blacks consuming high-fiber, low-fat, low-animal-product foods had virtually no risk of death from colon cancer, whereas the African whites consuming a low-fiber, high-fat diet had the same high risk as Westerners.

Animal fat, cholesterol, and meat protein have all been shown to have cancer-promoting properties in animal experiments and seem to increase the risk of colon polyps as well. Even chicken and fish have been found to be associated with high rates of colon cancer. The sulfur-containing amino acids found in high concentration in red meat, poultry, and fish produce large amounts of very noxious hydrogen sulfite, which has been shown to impair cellular metabolism and mucus production. Hydrogenated fats found in shortening, margarine, and many kinds of prepared and packaged foods may also be especially cancer-promoting. The guilty finger points clearly to meat, fat, and the lack of fruits, vegetables, and dietary fiber as the primary cause of polyps and subsequent colon cancer.

There have been many theories proposed regarding the effects of diet on cancer development. For example, a high-fat diet may increase the production of bile acids from the liver. In the colon, these bile acids are converted into cancer-causing substances by bowel bacteria. The kinds of bacteria that grow in the intestine depend upon the food we eat. On a rich diet, "unfriendly" bacteria flourish, making cancer-causing substances grow in the colon. It's a chain reaction set in motion with the first bite off the fork.

The Role of Dietary Fiber

Dietary fiber contributes to a healthy colon, and even overall health, by diluting and combining with cancer promoters in the bowel, thus reducing their access to the colon and the rest of our body. Fiber is also fermented into substances (like butyric acid) that inhibit the growth of cancer cells.

There are two general classes of fiber: *soluble and insoluble.* Wheat bran, which is classified as an insoluble fiber, appears to be the most effective at preventing colon disease, primarily by combining with and deactivating potentially harmful excess bile acids from the liver. Soluble fibers, such as guar gum, pectin, and oat bran, are less effective for colon cancer prevention but protect us more from heart disease and other diseases by decreasing cholesterol, improving insulin sensitivity, and reducing blood pressure.

One estimate suggests that if we were to increase our daily fiber intake by 13 grams, the risk of colon cancer would decrease by 31 percent—that's fifty thousand cases prevented in the United States annually! Another study, the Australian Polyp Prevention Project, found that a low-fat diet supplemented with wheat bran reduced the recurrence rate of large polyps (adenomas). So the good news is this—through dietary fiber nature has provided us with a most efficient mechanism for maintaining a healthy digestive system, and therefore a healthy body. Of course, you remember, dietary fiber is only found in plant foods. The bad news is the average American consumes a meager 8–14 grams of fiber a day.

Screening for Polyps and Colon Cancer

Since 1995, the United States Preventative Services Task Force, the American College of Physicians, the National Cancer Institute, the American Cancer Society, the World Health Organization, and the American Gastroenterological Association have been united in their recommendation that persons over the age of fifty with an average risk for colon cancer be screened through fecal occult blood tests, sigmoidoscopy, or both.

Unless there are special indications (such as a strong family history of colon cancer or a history of chronic colitis), I recommend one bowel exam between the ages of fifty-five and sixty years of age. If no polyps are detected, I recommend no future examinations. Why do I make such a recommendation? Since 90 percent of cancer occurs after the age of fifty-five, and the time required for transition from a normal colon to cancer is between twenty and thirty-five years, most cancers should be detected as polyps through a single screening between the age of fifty-five and sixty. Any polyps detected after this time would require longer than a typical life expectancy to transition from polyps to cancer.

While explaining to Larry the various diagnostic procedures, I noticed that he became visibly uneasy, an understandable reaction to the thought of having your private parts probed by complete strangers. I told Larry that my recommendation for him would be a double contrast barium enema and a sigmoid exam or a virtual colonoscopy by CT scan. Again, at the word colonoscopy, Larry became agitated.

I tried to offer some comfort. "I know these tests are not pleasant to think about, but I'm recommending the safest, most effective

Common Screening Methods

Digital Rectal Examination (DRE): Like most physical examination procedures, studies to date have shown DRE to be an ineffective diagnostic tool. By the time disease is detected through DRE, it will be at least ten years old, leaving limited options for treatment and recovery at this late stage.

Occult Blood Test: This is one of the most controversial areas of screening. Bleeding usually begins in the late stages of cancer, when a cure is unlikely. For every ten people who test positive for blood, one will be found to have cancer, four will have polyps, and five will be normal. These tests miss 20–50 percent of colon cancers and up to 80 percent of polyps. Besides its questionable effectiveness, fecal occult blood screening can lead to anxiety, loss of insurability, social stigma, and injury from any resulting tests and treatments.

Sigmoidoscopy Exam: In one often-cited study, screening through sigmoidoscopy every ten years reduced the risk of fatality from colorectal cancer by 55 percent. More frequent screening yielded no better results.

Optical Colonoscopy: Colonoscopy examination with a long flexible tube is called an optical colonoscopy. One reason most gastroenterologists encourage this diagnostic procedure is this procedure is one way they make their money—and as a result, most gastroenterologists are convinced that this money-making procedure is best for the patient. Besides monetary cost, this procedure requires intravenous administration of sedatives or a general anesthesia, and recovery time. Moreover, optical colonoscopy carries with it an inherent risk for bowel perforation, even when performed by the most skillful hands. Due to its invasive nature and the very real risk associated with optical colonoscopy, this procedure should be reserved for screening high-risk individuals and those who have previously been identified as having a polyp in need of removal.

Virtual Colonoscopy: This is the latest in high-tech detection using multiple CT-scanning X-rays. There are turf battles raging between medical specialists over which procedure is best, but one study in the *New England Journal of Medicine* reported this computer-based technique to be equal to or better than optical colonoscopy, and a much safer and less expensive screening tool for precancerous colon polyps. The procedure does cause discomfort, but most patients preferred the virtual rather than the optical colonoscopy. The virtual procedure takes about 14 minutes as compared to 32 minutes for the optical colonoscopy. One disadvantage of virtual colonoscopy (as well as the barium enema/sigmoidoscopy procedure) is that if a suspicious polyp is found, an optical colonoscopy must follow to remove the polyp. I prefer this procedure for an initial evaluation over optical colonoscopy.

(My preference) Sigmoid/Barium Enema: My preferred alternative to either kind of colonoscopy is a time-honored double-contrast barium enema and a flexible sigmoidoscope, which is much lower in cost with fewer complications. Optical colonoscopy examinations, performed by experienced specialists, miss finding polyps 24 percent of the time, and they are much more dangerous and costly than a barium enema and a sigmoid examination. Virtual colonoscopy exams are costly too. Unfortunately, strong bias among doctors will keep this information away from you.

procedures for your situation. I'll be sending you to the best specialists I know. You'll be in good hands."

"I know you know what you're doing, Dr. McDougall, It's just that my best friend, Dave, on the bowling team, had a colonoscopy done, and the doctor perforated his colon. Dave spent a week in ICU and almost died. Then he spent two more weeks in the hospital on IV antibiotics and getting poked and prodded so they could fix the screwup. They told him he'll probably have to be tested for the rest of his life to make sure the patch job is holding up."

No wonder Larry had such a reaction to my recommendation. "Larry," I assured him, "I completely understand your apprehension given your friend's nightmare."

Powerful Medicine for Colon Disease

Present-day treatment of colon cancer—surgery, radiation, and/or chemotherapy—does little to reduce a person's risk of dying of this disease. Even surgical removal of polyps before they transition into cancerous growths proves ineffective, because eventually new ones take their place. Interestingly, polyps have been shown to regress and disappear when fecal material is diverted away from the colon by surgical colostomy. How does this happen? Remember the analogy of the callused hand? Just like the callus in the palm of the hand softens and disappears when hard work ends, polyps can also disappear when the toxic irritation of harmful foods (via fecal matter) is removed from the colon.

Can a person who already has colon cancer benefit from a healthful diet? There is substantial evidence that a low-fat, no cholesterol diet can slow the growth of cancer and allow a person to live a longer, healthier life. In very rare cases people have recovered from colon cancer—this is called spontaneous remission.

The most significant recommendation being withheld from patients suffering from any form of colon disease is this—Stop throwing gasoline on the fire! Without a change in lifestyle, the cause of irritation and ultimately disease is ever-present. By adopting a healthful plant-based diet low in fat, such as the McDougall Diet, individuals battling polyps, colon cancer, and all other intestinal troubles will begin to implement the most powerful weapon at their disposal.

Larry Gets a Second Chance

Following Larry's tests, he and Louise returned to my office to hear the results. Thankfully I had good news to deliver. Larry's tests turned out the way we'd hoped—no polyps, no cancer. All we found was hemorrhoids—the source of the blood Larry saw in the toilet. Because of Larry's chronic constipation, his hemorrhoids had worsened to the point of more frequent and pronounced bleeding. As for the cramps, we learned that Larry's stomach was adamantly protesting his penchant for pork.

Louise squeezed Larry's hand and kissed him on the cheek. Larry responded with relief, "Whew, I'll take hemorrhoids over cancer any day."

"You don't have to," I said. "When you start eating the foods Louise is eating, and I mean for more than a week, you'll most likely find relief from your hemorrhoids and your constant gut ache. On the McDougall Diet you'll consume a whopping 40–100 grams of fiber a day, enough to keep you happy and regular and free of troublesome hemorrhoids."

Recalling with Larry what his life had been like for years strengthened his determination to stop damaging his body and get back on the road to health. He had wasted countless hours straining to produce a paltry bowel movement every few days, which even then brought only minimal relief. Then the pendulum would swing and he'd spend the next days or weeks suffering from cramps and diarrhea, worried he wouldn't be able to find a bathroom if the urge struck in public. He admitted living with the fear that all his distresses might eventually lead to a life-threatening illness like colon cancer. Larry's health struggles had affected his ability to focus at work and had forced him to use more sick days than he cared to count. But Larry's deepest regrets surrounded the family times he'd forfeited because of his health issues. He'd missed his seven-year-old granddaughter's winning field goal in her first soccer game of the season. He'd missed his grandson's birthday party— an all games and miniature golf. He'd wanted to take Louise out to a nice restaurant for her fiftieth birthday, but when the big day arrived, so did severe, stabbing abdominal cramps. They stayed home and had chicken broth with crackers.

Larry was finally figuring out that it's far easier to adapt once and for all to a new, healthful way of eating than it is to continually adapt to whatever physical ailment strikes next. This time he was ready to make healthful eating a permanent part of his life. He knew how much he had to lose if he didn't, and more importantly, how much he had to gain if he did.

Before leaving, Larry said sincerely, "This time I'm going to do it, Doc. I'm sick of being sick."

I responded, "I know you will, Larry. Next time I see you I expect to hear lots of good news."

He added with a grin, "And lots of stories about adventures with my grandkids."

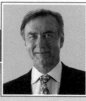

SUMMARY SHEET *from Dr. McDougall*

- *A person over fifty years of age has about a 5 percent lifetime chance of developing colon cancer.*

- *Colon cancer arises from polyps—35 percent of people consuming the typical Western diet are found to have colon polyps.*

- *Polyps take an average of fifteen years to turn into cancer—the bigger they are in size, the further along they are on this terrible journey.*

- *The whole process from normal colon cells to cancer and death will span, on average, twenty to thirty-five years.*

- *The risk (or lack thereof) for colon cancer is passed from generation to generation when parents teach sons and daughters how to cook and what foods to enjoy.*

- *Meat, fat, and the lack of fruits, vegetables, and dietary fiber is the primary cause of polyps and subsequent colon cancer.*

- *I recommend one bowel exam between fifty-five and sixty years of age, and no subsequent examinations if polyps are not present.*

- *The preferred mode of screening for polyps is a double-contrast barium enema and a flexible sigmoidoscope, or a virtual colonoscopy—one time at approximately sixty years of age.*

- *A key component of polyp therapy is removal of the root cause— offensive foods that irritate the lining of the colon.*

- *A healthful, low-fat, no cholesterol diet may slow the growth of cancer and allow a person to live a longer, healthier life.*

CHAPTER 12

Beneficial Bowel Bacteria

L arry and Louise were surprised and a bit skeptical when I told them one of our goals was to make their intestines a breeding ground for bacteria—good bacteria that is. Like most folks in our antibacterial, sterile society, the Bortons believed all bacteria were bad and should certainly be banned from entering the body. As I explained to this disbelieving couple, the vast majority of bacterial organisms are actually helpful, or at least not harmful, to our lives.

"Should I stop cleaning the house, Doc?" asked Louise. "Because I'd certainly make that sacrifice for my health and the health of my dear husband."

"I know you would, Louise," I responded. "But that's not the kind of bacteria I'm talking about. It's awfully generous of you to offer though."

I began to explain to the Bortons what I meant by healthful, or good, bacteria, and how keeping this bacteria flourishing in their bodies would help them achieve and maintain the good health they deserved and had been lacking for more years than they could remember.

Within our intestines live trillions of organisms that are so important to our health and survival that they should be thought of as a vital organ—just like our livers or kidneys. The *gut microflora* is the name we give to this living factory, whose beneficial functions include: completing the digestion of our foods through fermenta-

117

tion, protecting us against disease-causing microbes, synthesizing water-soluble vitamins, and stimulating the development and function of our immune systems.

Our intestinal tracts contain a complex and diverse society of disease-causing (pathogenic) and "friendly" bacteria. Rule number one is simple: dominance by the "good guys" will crowd out and leave no room in our intestines for the "bad guys." In addition to digesting remnants of our meals and synthesizing vitamins, the helpful bacteria play an important role in the development of the immune system by maintaining a constant dialogue with our internal bodies through the surface of the gut. Our microflora also influence many of our hormones. The health consequences from an imbalance of our sex hormones can lead to precocious puberty, fibrocystic breast disease, PMS, uterine fibroids, prostate enlargement, and breast, uterine, and prostate cancer. When our bowel bacteria really get out of control, severe forms of colitis and colon cancer can be the consequences.

The Microbial Factory

Bacteria are not distributed randomly throughout the intestinal tract but are found in different numbers and kinds in different regions of the gut. The mouth provides a fertile garden for millions of bacteria, but the stomach (because of the acid) and small intestine contain a very low level of bacteria. The final five feet of the intestine, known as the large intestine or colon, works as a microbial factory, with more than five hundred different species of bacteria living in a three-pound (1.5 kg) mass of partially digested matter. Within the colon the concentration of bacteria reaches one trillion organisms per gram (1/30th of an ounce) of feces. Bacteria make up about 60 percent of the weight of the feces. The microflora are so important to our well-being that after a person's colon is surgically removed (colectomy), the last part of the small intestine (ilium) takes over this vital role and becomes colonized with a similar biomass of bacteria.

The health of the flora can become impaired by temperature, illnesses, antibiotics and other drug treatments, and changes in our

Benefits of a Healthy Gut Microflora

- Increase the natural resistance to infections from bacteria, yeast, and viruses.
- Prevent traveler's diarrhea.
- Speed healing from diarrheal diseases and relapsing colitis.
- Improve digestion.
- Relieve constipation.
- Stimulate the immune system.
- Lessen symptoms of inflammatory arthritis.
- Suppress cancer development and growth.
- Reduce sex hormones.
- Reduce cholesterol and triglycerides.

diets. The effects of antibiotic therapy can be profound and persistent, even causing a life-threatening infection with overgrowth of pathogenic bacteria (called *Clostridium difficile*).

The Beginnings of Good Bacteria

Before birth, the gastrointestinal tract of a normal fetus is sterile. When the newborn passes through the birth canal, he or she is thoroughly inoculated with organisms from the mother's vagina and bowel. Benefits to the infant begin immediately with this natural defense barrier of "friendly" bacteria standing against harmful microbes that will enter later on with touching, suckling, kissing, and caressing.

The importance of this early invasion of friendly bacteria should not be underestimated. Its presence or absence makes a permanent impression on the immune system, thereby affecting a person's well-being throughout his or her life. Newborns delivered by cesarean section do not get a healthful dose of the mother's bacteria. Born through the abdomen, much of their initial bacteria come from the unhygienic environment of a hospital. However, this setback can be remedied by the initiation of proper infant feeding after birth—and boosted by the addition of infant probiotics (see below).

Breast-feeding encourages the growth of "friendly" bacteria known as *Bifidobacterium*. These vital organisms protect the baby from gastrointestinal infections that can result in illnesses severe enough to require hospitalization and sometimes cause death. Mother's milk contains sugars (galactooligosaccharides) that encourage the growth of these friendly bacteria. By the fourth day of life, *Bifidobacterium* represent 48 percent of the bacteria in breast-fed infants as opposed to 15 percent in bottle-fed infants. Eventually, over 95 percent of the bacteria become *Bifidobacterium* bacteria in an exclusively breast-fed baby. Introduction of small amounts of formula to a breast-fed baby will result in shifts from a breast-fed to a formula-fed pattern of the microflora. After weaning from breast milk—ideally after the age of two years—the child's flora becomes similar to an adult's.

Healthful Diet Equals Healthy Microflora

How do healthy microflora thrive? The microflora in our large intestines thrive on the partially digested remnants of our meals—they eat what we eat. The microflora require approximately 250 calories of carbohydrate daily just to survive. Each species of bacteria survives best on specific kinds of nutrients. In short, friendly bacteria prefer dining on plant-food remnants, and pathogens prefer eating meat and other "junk-food." Therefore, what we choose to eat determines the predominance of the bacteria species that will live in our gut—friendly or pathogenic. By eating a diet based on whole plant foods rather than on animal foods and highly processed foods, you can suppress the growth of harmful bacteria and stimulate the growth of those that are beneficial. If your current diet is one that feeds the pathogenic bacteria, take heart. Major alterations in the microflora take place within one to two weeks of a healthful diet change.

Bacteria enjoy the parts of the plant foods that we don't use. Undigestible complex carbohydrates (dietary fiber) and other smaller undigestible sugars (oligosaccharides) provide the bulk of the food for our bowel bacteria. Only plants contain these complex and simple carbohydrates (except for breast milk, as noted above). These undigestible simple sugars are abundant in artichokes, onions, chicory, garlic, leeks, and, to a lesser extent, cereals. Beans, peas, and lentils contain the oligosaccharides raffinose and stachyose that feed our friendly bowel bacteria. Purified wood cellulose, which has been used to manufacture some "high-fiber breads," is not broken down by the microflora. Because only plants contain these microflora-nourishing sugars, strict vegetarians (vegans) have been found to harbor much higher counts of "friendly" bacteria than do meat-eaters.

Manipulating Our Microflora with Probiotic Supplements

The buzzword "probiotics" will be popping up more and more as health-conscious individuals become increasingly aware of the role of gut microflora. Probiotics are used for the purpose of adding a particular species of bacteria in order to rebalance the intestines and thereby improve a person's health. Probiotics are sold as foods and pills (supplements) that contain millions of friendly bacteria and sometimes yeast. Purchased in natural food stores, probiotics are usually found in the refrigerated section. Some are labeled as "newborn formulas," while others are aimed at improving the flora of a child or an adult. Probiotics have no toxic effects.

Prebiotics and Synbiotics

Prebiotics are nondigestible simple sugars (oligosaccharides) sold as pills and liquids that stimulate the growth and/or activity of friendly bacteria *already present* in our intestines. Prebiotics are very effective for relieving constipation and hold some promise for the prevention of gallstones as well as for the treatment of inflammatory bowel diseases. Examples of undigestible sugars used as prebiotics

Conditions Aided by Specific Probiotics

Used as single agents or in combinations

Dental Caries:
 Lactobacillus rhamnosus
H. Pylori (Stomach Ulcer):
 Lactobacillus johnsonii
 Lactobacillus paracasei
Acute and Chronic Diarrhea:
 Lactobacillus acidophilus
 Lactobacillus casei
 Lactobacillus reuteri
 Lactobacillus rhamnosus (GG)
 Bifidobacteria bifidum
Irritable Bowel Syndrome:
 Lactobacillus acidophilus
 Lactobacillus plantarum
Lactose Intolerance:
 Lactobacillus acidophilus
 Lactobacillus bulgaricus
 Bifidobacteria longum
Constipation:
 Lactobacillus casei
 Lactobacillus reuteri
 Lactobacillus rhamnosus
 Bifidobacteria animals
 Saccharomyces cerevisiae (yeast)
 Propionibacterium freudenreichii
Crohn's Disease:
 Lactobacillus rhamnosus (GG)
 Saccharomyces boulardii
 Escherichia coli, Nissle strain (1917)
Ulcerative Colitis:
 Escherichia coli, Nissle strain (1917)
 BIFICO (3 Bifidobacteria species)
 Saccharomyces boulardii
 VLS 3 brand (Lactobacillus and
   Bifidobacteria)

Diverticular Disease of Colon:
 Escherichia coli, Nissle strain (1917)
Vaginal Candida:
 Lactobacillus acidophilus
 Lactobacillus rhamnosus
 Lactobacillus fermentum
Elevated Cholesterol:
 Lactobacillus acidophilus
 Lactobacillus bulgaricus
 Lactobacillus plantarum
 Streptococcus thermophilus
 Enterococcus faecium
Elevated Blood Sugar (diabetes):
 Saccharomyces cerevisiae (yeast)
Rheumatoid Arthritis:
 Lactobacillus rhamnosus
Eczema (atopic dermatitis):
 Bifidobacteria lactis
 Streptococcus thermophilus
 Lactobacillus rhamnosus
Premenstrual Syndrome:
 Saccharomyces cerevisiae (yeast)
General Immunity:
 Lactobacillus plantarum
 Lactobacillus johnsonii
 Lactobacillus rhamnosus
 Bifidobacteria lactis
 Bifidobacteria bifidum
 Escherichia coli, Nissle strain (1917)
Growth or Weight of Infants:
 Bifidobacteria bifidum
 Bifidobacteria breve
 Streptococcus thermophilus
Colon Cancer Prevention:
 Bifidobacterium

are: FOS (fructooligosaccharides), GOS (galactooligosaccharides), inulin (not insulin), lactulose, and lactitol. Two prebiotics prescribed by doctors, lactulose and lactitol, have been effectively used to treat patients with liver failure (hepatic encephalopathy). They may also be helpful in the prevention of colon cancer.

These commercial prebiotics, just like probiotics, have no toxic effects. They can act as a mild laxative in small amounts, but may produce flatulence when consumed in large amounts. Combining probiotics (the bacteria) with prebiotics (the bacteria's food) results in a logical partnership called *synbiotics*. You will most often find synbiotic products sold as mixtures of bacteria with FOS (fructooligosaccharides). Because the McDougall Diet is comprised of starches, vegetables, and fruits that contain a wide variety of undigestible sugars that feed and stimulate the growth of "friendly" bacteria, people consuming such a diet require no additional prebiotics. Their microflora are healthy and flourishing as they feast on the remnants of healthful, plant-based meals.

Dairy as a Probiotic Source

The best-known examples of food containing probiotics are yogurts containing lactic-acid-producing bacteria called *Lactobacillus bulgaricus.* These organisms are nontoxic and survive passage through the intestine. However, they cannot live and reproduce in the colon (they do not colonize the colon); therefore, they must be ingested regularly for any health-promoting properties to persist. I do not recommend yogurt as a source of friendly bacteria for two reasons. First, these bacteria's beneficial effects have not been conclusively proven. Second, and more importantly, yogurt brings with it all the negative qualities of dairy products: high fat and cholesterol content, allergy-producing dairy proteins, and potential infection with harmful viruses and bacteria. Acidophilus milk is made by culturing milk with Lactobacillus acidophilus bacteria and has similar drawbacks. Any benefits of Lactobacillus can be obtained much more safely and effectively in supplement forms (pills), thereby avoiding the health risks of dairy products.

Who Needs Healthy Gut Bacteria?

A healthy microflora is necessary for overall health—period. Anyone who wants to be healthy should encourage the growth of healthy microflora by eating the right foods and avoiding antibiotics (which kill both good and bad bacteria) whenever possible. This means a "breast-milk diet" for infants and a healthful plant-based diet (like the McDougall Diet) for children and adults.

Newborns delivered by cesarean section and bottle-fed babies may benefit from probiotics specifically designed for infant use. Probiotics may also be warranted after a course of prescribed antibiotics in order to help reestablish a healthy gut flora. Probiotic supplements, in addition, may prove beneficial if you have changed your diet and still suffer from problems such as irregular bowel movements, indigestion, elevated cholesterol, or arthritis. With no undesirable side effects and minimal cost, you have everything to gain and nothing to lose by trying probiotic supplements.

For Larry and Louise, we found that a simple diet change brought about the desired results, so no added probiotic supplements were necessary. I've seen this happen over and over in my practice. That is why I am convinced that a healthful plant-based diet is the fuel our bodies were made to thrive on . . . friendly bacteria and all.

SUMMARY SHEET *from Dr. McDougall*

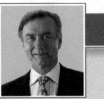

- *The gut microflora is the name we give to the vital living factory of bacteria living within our colons.*

- *The microflora complete digestion of foods, protect us against pathogens, synthesize vitamins, reduce cholesterol, balance hormones, and stimulate our immune systems.*

- *Breast-feeding encourages the growth of "friendly" bacteria known as Bifidobacterium.*

- *"Friendly" bacteria prefer dining on plant-food remnants, and pathogens prefer eating meat and other "junk-food."*

- *Dietary fiber and other smaller undigestible sugars, all from plants, provide the bulk of the food for our bowel bacteria.*

- *Probiotics add bacteria to the bowel in order to rebalance the intestines and thereby improve a person's health.*

- *Specific species of bacteria must be used in order to target specific health concerns.*

- *Prebiotics are simple sugar foods sold as pills and liquids that stimulate the growth and/or activity of friendly bacteria already present in our intestines.*

- *A healthful diet provides excellent foods for the microflora, so no additional prebiotics are required.*

- *Dairy foods (yogurt and acidophilus) are unhealthful sources of probiotics.*

- *Probiotics are beneficial for people still suffering with problems such as irregular bowel movements, indigestion, elevated cholesterol, or arthritis, even after a healthful change in diet.*

CHAPTER 13

Flatulence

EXPLORING THE F-WORD

Y ou'll recall how pleased the Bortons were when we first met to learn how their new way of eating would help eliminate bad breath. Louise was quick to express concern at that time about an odor of a different kind.

"Dr. McDougall, Larry seems to have some issues with smells a little farther south. Can your diet do anything about that?"

My answer regarding Larry's excess smelly gas wasn't quite what Louise or Larry expected. They were puzzled initially by what I had to say but stuck with me for the happy ending.

"Larry and Louise, you've heard the term flatulence?"

Larry responded, "Isn't that a two-dollar word for farts or passing gas?" Louise administered a firm nudge to the ribs.

"Yes, that's right, Larry. The word flatulence comes from the term flatus, meaning intestinal gas. The average person on the typical American diet passes gas ten to twenty times a day with an average daily volume of 705 ml—that's over 20 ounces or about a quart and a half of gas, if you want the details."

"See there, Larry, I knew you were above average," Louise contributed. "So what's the least amount of gas one can pass?"

Louise was surprised to hear that, by contrast, individuals on a liquid diet devoid of all complex sugars have been found to pass gas an average of 1.5 times in twenty-four hours with a total volume of only 214 ml—or about 7 ounces. They were just as surprised to find that someone actually studies flatulence.

The major gas source for most people is the bacterial activity within the colon as it works to complete digestion of our foods. The carbohydrates that our small intestine is unable to break down move on to the large intestine (colon), where they are broken down by bacteria through a process of fermentation. These indigestible carbohydrates—as opposed to the ones our intestines *can* break down and use for energy—are also known as *dietary fiber,* or simply referred to as "fiber" in our foods. The result of this fermenting in the intestine is a gaseous mixture consisting primarily of nitrogen (N_2), oxygen (O_2), carbon dioxide (CO_2), hydrogen (H_2), and methane (CH_4). These gases are all odorless and colorless.

Stinky gas (the kind that smells like rotten eggs) is caused by sulfur-producing foods. So which foods produce the most sulfur? An experiment on five healthy men on five different diets for ten days each showed that over fifteen times more sulfur was produced with the meat diet than with the vegetarian diet. Except for garlic, broccoli, and cauliflower, most vegetables are low in sulfur.

The most common source of undigested carbohydrates in the American diet, and therefore the leading cause of excess gas, is lactose from dairy products, such as milk, skim milk, and yogurt (cheeses contain little lactose). Dairy foods, including cheese, also contain large amounts of stinky sulfur. Larry was quick to point out that this may be the origin of the common phrase "cutting the cheese" when someone passes noticeable gas. This bit of insight prompted another nudge to the ribs from Louise.

All unrefined plant foods, including grains, fruits, and vegetables, contain indigestible carbohydrates that end up being fermented in the large intestine and are expelled as gases. Refining grains into white flour and rice removes most of the indigestible carbohydrates (dietary fiber). White rice is one complex carbohydrate that is almost completely absorbed by the small intestine, resulting in very little indigestible carbohydrate for bacteria in the colon to turn into flatus.

When Louise eagerly suggested that she'd be happy to cook white rice for Larry—breakfast, lunch, and dinner—I couldn't resist sharing an interesting bit of information I'd read just the previous week. In a scientific experiment on flatus (yes, you read that correctly), odor was rated from 0 (no odor) to 8 (very offensive) by the highly trained noses of two distinguished judges. No, really, I'm serious. Women were rated with an average score of 5.45 and men with an average score of 3.95 on the offensiveness scale. However, men passed higher volumes of gas than did women (119 ml vs. 88 ml per passage).

Louise interjected, "Well, that proves it, Dr. McDougall. Men really *are* full of hot air." Larry and I decided it best to leave that one alone.

Creating a Gas Shortage

From the moment Louise mentioned Larry's gas problem, I had a strong hunch about his daily diet. Sure enough, a brief survey confirmed my suspicions. For Larry, a meal was not complete without a big hunk of meat, preferably pork, plopped down in the middle of the plate, and a jumbo glass of milk to wash it down; his bedtime ritual included a nightly behemoth bowl of ice cream. By consuming massive quantities of gaseous dairy products with sulfur-rich meat to boot, Larry had perfected the formula for stinky gas, and lots of it.

Larry and Louise were relieved to learn that they are not powerless when it comes to controlling the gas they pass. However, I gave the Bortons some helpful suggestions to help eliminate excess gas and reduce the offensive odors.

Enjoy a Vegetarian Diet

By limiting intake of sulfur-producing foods, you can greatly reduce the amount of offensive gas you pass. With the elimination of all animal products, which are the major sulfur producers, the primary source of the offensive odors is removed. This repulsive smell should be telling you that there is something wrong within your bowel, and, it follows, something unhealthful for your body. In

Chapter 3, in the section on halitosis (page 11), I explained that foul-smelling sulfur is associated with more heart disease, cancer, severe forms of colitis, and risk of earlier death. A sure sign that you are a healthier person will be communicated to you and close friends by your improvement in body odors.

You should be aware that in the first few days of your new plant-based, high-fiber diet, you will seem to produce more gas than before; however, your body will adjust to this new way of eating, and the amount of gas produced should diminish within about two weeks. Much of this adjustment comes as a result of changes in the kinds and numbers of bacteria present in the bowel, the gut microflora we discussed earlier. Though you may experience this temporary increase in gas production, the knowledge that your new dietary choices can relieve virtually all your digestive difficulties, as well as help you avoid cancer and heart disease, makes it worth a little extra gas.

Avoid Gassy Foods

Milk products are very troublesome, especially for most non-Caucasian people (Asians, Blacks, Hispanics, Indians, Eskimos) who can't digest lactose, although about 20 percent of Caucasians also experience lactose intolerance. Legumes (beans, peas, and lentils) contain two relatively indigestible sugars called raffinose and stachyose, making them the second-leading producers of excess gas. If you don't want the extra gas but are afraid you won't get enough protein without beans, don't worry. All the protein you need is readily available in the other less gassy starches and vegetables that abound in the McDougall Diet.

Some individuals experience troublesome gas production from onions, bagels, pretzels, prunes, apricots, cabbage, carrots, celery, green peppers, broccoli, cauliflower, bananas, Brussels sprouts, and wheat germ. This list of offenders is highly dependent on personal sensitivities, so any number of foods could be included. By paying attention to the foods you eat and your patterns of gas production, you will soon be able to pinpoint and eliminate the guilty excess gas producers.

Cooking Methods Can Help

Almost everyone seems to have a method of "degassing" beans. Some say, "Add potatoes to beans during cooking," or "Discard the rinse water after soaking beans." The truth is, soaking itself does help by starting the breakdown of the carbohydrates—but this benefit has nothing to do with discarding the rinse water. Cooking does break down many of the gas-forming complex carbohydrates found in most grains and vegetables. In legumes, however, the indigestible sugars (raffinose and stachyose) are heat-stable and resistant to cooking.

There is one reliable way to "degas" beans—sprouting. To sprout beans before cooking, simply cover the beans with water for twelve hours, drain off the water, then spread out the beans on a damp paper towel, and let them sit for another twelve hours. When you notice tiny white shoots (one-sixteenth inch long) beginning to appear, it means the little plant has utilized most of the indigestible sugars for growth. Your beans are now ready to cook. Cooking time will be greatly reduced after the sprouting process—and so will your gassiness.

Beano

This product, available at supermarkets, natural foods stores, and drugstores in the form of liquid drops and tablets, contains enzymes that are capable of breaking down the indigestible sugars in beans, peas, lentils, and other gaseous vegetables. The Beano label claims that if you add one or two drops with the first bite of food, you'll be able to enjoy the rest of your meal with no gas worries. (Beano contains fish derived enzymes; strict vegetarians may choose other similar capsules made without animal-derived ingredients.)

Activated Charcoal

Although activated charcoal has been used to treat intestinal gas in India and Europe for many years, only recently has it begun gaining acceptance in the United States. In laboratory studies, activated charcoal was found to bind and deactivate sulfur gases. However, its efficacy as demonstrated in human studies remains questionable.

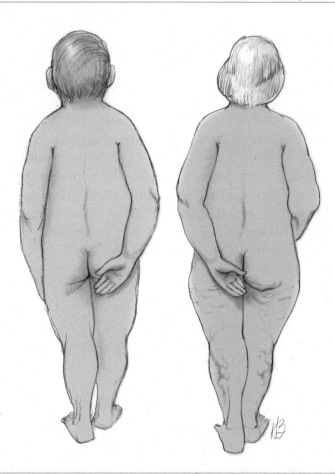

What's a little gas among friends? Certainly a small inconvenience for great health and good looks.

Probiotics

A change in the kinds of bacteria in the large intestine—the intestinal microflora—can result in reduced flatulence. Probiotics contain the kinds of bacteria necessary to achieve a healthy balance of microflora. In a controlled study, volunteers with irritable bowel syndrome (IBS) were fed a probiotic drink containing *Lactobacillus plantarum*, a friendly form of bowel bacteria, for four weeks. Flatulence was rapidly and significantly reduced in the test group as compared with the placebo group.

Avoid Unnecessary Medications

Many medications are known to cause flatulence, so this is something to consider if you notice increased gas problems after starting a new medication. Two common medications that can cause gassiness by increasing sugars in the large intestine are acarbose for diabetes and lactulose for constipation.

The Bortons Get Gas—The Good Kind

Just as I suspected, a couple of days into their new dietary program, Louise phoned my office. "Dr. McDougall, something's wrong. Larry is noisier than ever, and now I'm talking when I walk too. No offense, Dr. McDougall, but it's so noticeable, Larry's been joking, 'Hey, heard a good McBugle lately?'"

"No offense taken," I chuckled. "Louise, remember I said that at first you may have even more gas than usual but it would improve dramatically after your body becomes used to this new, more healthful way of eating." A week after her frantic phone call, Louise left a message on my machine, "I can't believe it, Dr. McDougall. I no longer have to run for cover every time Larry, well, you know. And the 'McBugle' jokes are pretty much over. Thanks a million."

SUMMARY SHEET *from Dr. McDougall*

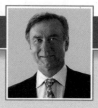

- *Passing gas is a normal, natural part of life.*
- *In general, the more flatus, the more healthful the diet.*
- *The major source of gas is from bacterial activity working to digest the remnants of the food.*
- *Fermentation of carbohydrates produces odorless gasses: nitrogen, oxygen, carbon dioxide, hydrogen, and methane.*
- *The most common source of undigested carbohydrates, and therefore troublesome gas, is the milk sugar lactose, from dairy products.*
- *Two undigestible sugars, raffinose and stachyose, found in beans, are notorious sources of gas.*
- *Foul odors are from putrefaction and the release of sulfur compounds.*
- *Offensive flatus is an important indication of something wrong inside your body.*
- *Dietary derived sulfur is involved in the cause of heart disease, cancer, colitis, and death.*
- *Thorough cooking and sprouting are effective degassing methods.*
- *If excess gas from beans bothers you, then eliminate them—there is ample protein in all other unprocessed starch and green and yellow vegetable foods to meet your needs.*
- *Beano is very effective for reducing gas.*
- *As strange as this may sound, inoffensive smelling bowel gas is a sign of good health.*

CHAPTER 14

Evolution, Anatomy, and Proper Human Nutrition

When the Bortons came in for a follow-up appointment six months after Larry's final pledge to stick to a healthful diet, they both reported positive progress with regard to all their health issues. They were feeling better than ever and expressed only one concern. Louise explained.

"Dr. McDougall, even though our kids see how well we're doing, they don't seem to think this way of eating is for them. Now that we know the truth about what's good for us, we want our kids and grandkids to eat healthfully too."

Larry added, "I know they sincerely want the best for their kids, but it breaks my heart to hear them say, 'Finish your cheeseburger, honey. It's good for you.' What can we do to convince them they should be eating differently if they want to stay healthy?"

Larry describes a scenario that is played out in households across the nation every day. I personally knew the drill only too well. "Johnny, eat your meat. You need your protein." With only the best intentions for her growing child, my mother repeated this mantra at almost every meal. "But Mom, I can't chew it," I tried to explain. To appease her worry over my health, I mashed the bite-sized hunk of roast beef with my teeth into a leathery lump, still too big to comfortably swallow. Eventually, jaw-tired and wanting to be excused from the table, I slipped the remains under the edge of my plate.

Conscientious parents urge their children to eat their meat so they can grow big and strong. Children labor to the point of frustration to chew up the hunks of "nutrition" on their plates. I firmly believe that if well-meaning parents, just like Larry and Louise, were simply exposed to the truth about proper human nutrition, much of this distress could be avoided. I gave them the following information to pass on to their grown children in hopes that it would have a positive influence on their ideas about which foods really are good for us.

What Evolution Says about Nutrition

E volution in the animal kingdom dates back hundreds of millions of years, with the development of upright-standing humanoids beginning over four million years ago. The ancestors of modern humans were believed to live almost exclusively on plant foods—wild fruits, leaves, roots, and other high-quality plant parts—with very few animal foods in their daily diet. These prehumans ate like our nearest primate relatives, the apes of today.

Biologists at Wayne State University School of Medicine in Detroit, Michigan, provide new genetic evidence that lineages of chimpanzees and humans diverged so recently that chimps should be reclassified as members of our genus *Homo,* along with Neanderthals and all other human-like fossil species. "We humans appear as only slightly remodeled chimpanzee-like apes," say these researchers. A recent publication in the journal *Nature* reported that of the 3 billion genes that make up humans and chimpanzees, 96 percent are identical—demonstrating our genetic similarity. Our common genetic ancestor of six million years ago undoubtedly lived primarily on a vegetarian diet, as we should.

Given this connection between humans and our closest relatives, the apes, let's look at the dietary makeup of these primates. Most apes living today eat essentially as vegetarians. They consume a diet of fruits, leaves, flowers, and bark, with sporadic consumption of very small amounts of insect material (like termites) and, less commonly, small animals. Our anatomical and physiological features, so closely resembling those of the chimpanzee, are clear indicators of the types of foods that should comprise our diet today.

What Anatomy Says about Nutrition

O ur teeth are designed for processing starches, fruits, and vegetables—not for tearing and chewing flesh. What many refer to as our "canine teeth" are nothing at all like the sharp blades of true carnivores designed for processing meat. I lecture to over ten thousand dentists, dental hygienists, and oral specialists every year, and I always ask them to show me the "canine" teeth in a person's mouth (those that resemble a cat's or a dog's teeth). I have yet to be shown the first example of a sharply pointed, true canine tooth belonging to a person.

The lower jaw of a meat-eating animal has very little capacity for side-to-side motion. It is fixed only to open and close, which adds strength and stability to its powerful bite. Like those of other plant-eating animals, the human jaw can open and close as well as move forward and backward and side-to-side. This is an ideal range of motion for biting off pieces of plant matter and then grinding them into smaller pieces with our flat molars. Because of our inadequate ability to chew and swallow meat, choking is a common occurrence in populations consuming a typical Western diet. Approximately four thousand people die each year in the United States from choking on food, usually meat products—a condition referred to as a "café coronary."

On the tips of our tongues are sensors that are designed to seek out sweet-tasting foods—carbohydrates (sugars). While plant foods are loaded with carbohydrates, there are essentially none of these sweet-tasting substances in red meat, poultry, fish, shellfish, eggs, or cheese. By contrast, the tongue of a carnivore does not have sensors for carbohydrates; instead, carnivores have taste buds that are pleasantly stimulated by animal proteins (aminos). Omnivores, like dogs, have retained taste buds for both proteins and sugars.

What Our Digestive System Says about Nutrition

F rom top to bottom, our digestive system has evolved to efficiently process plant foods. Digestion begins in the mouth with a salivary enzyme called alpha-amylase (ptyalin), whose sole purpose is to help break down complex carbohydrates from plant foods into simple sugars. There are no carbohydrates in meats of any kind (except for a smidgen of glycogen), so a true carnivore has no need for this enzyme—their salivary glands do not synthesize alpha-amylase.

The stomach juices of a meat-eating animal are very concentrated in acid in order to efficiently break down the large quantities of muscle and bone materials ingested by these carnivores. In people and other plant-eaters, digestion of starches, vegetables, and fruits is accomplished efficiently with much lower concentrations of stomach acid.

The human intestine is long and coiled, much like that of apes, cows, and horses. This configuration makes digestion slow, allowing time to break down and absorb the nutrients from plant foods. The intestine of a carnivore, like a cat, is short, straight, and tubular. This allows for very rapid digestion of flesh and excretion of the remnants quickly, before they putrefy (rot). There are also marked sacculations (many sac-like enlargements that bulge out along our large intestine), like those found in all apes, which strongly support the view that we are primarily plant-eating animals. Overall, the intestines of meat-eaters are noticeably simpler than those of plant-eaters like you and me.

Cholesterol Overwhelms a Plant-Eater's Liver

It is no secret that cholesterol is harmful to the human body. What is not widely known is that cholesterol is found only in animal foods—not a bit in plant foods. The liver and biliary system of a meat-eating animal has an unlimited capacity to process and excrete cholesterol from its body. For example, you can feed a dog or cat pure egg yolks all day long, and they will excrete all of it, never suffering from a buildup of cholesterol. On the other hand, humans (like other plant-eating animals) have livers with very limited capacities for cholesterol removal. As a result, most people have great difficulty eliminating the amounts of cholesterol they take in from eating animal products.

What appears to be an "inefficiency" of our livers is actually a result of our evolutionary design. We were made to consume plant foods (containing no cholesterol); therefore, we have never required a highly efficient cholesterol-eliminating biliary system.

The resulting cholesterol buildup from eating red meat, poultry, fish, shellfish, eggs, and dairy foods causes deposits to form in the arteries (atherosclerosis) as well as in the skin under the eyes (xanthelasma) and in the tendons. Bile supersaturated with cholesterol forms gallstones (over 95 percent of gallstones are made of cholesterol), a condition that affects about half of all middle-aged women who consume a typical Western diet.

Our Bodies Need Plant Nutrients

itamins are essential micronutrients that *cannot* be synthesized by the body and must be obtained in the food we consume. Since plants, plentiful in vitamin C (ascorbic acid), have always been a reliable part of our diet, we have lost the ability to synthesize (make our own) ascorbic acid. Thus this substance is a necessary nutrient—vitamin—for humans. Because ascorbic acid has *not* been reliably available to primarily meat-eating animals, they have retained the ability to manufacture their own ascorbic acid from the basic raw materials found in their meat diet. This is just one of many examples of the metabolic processes and nutritional needs that clearly say our bodies are designed to thrive on a diet of plant foods.

Our Instincts Are for Plants

While many individuals react adversely to the thought of consuming fresh meat (especially something unfamiliar, such as kangaroo, rat, or cat), most do not have a negative reaction to any fruits and vegetables, even when unfamiliar. Imagine if I were to ask you to try an unknown "star fruit" from the tropics for the first time. You would try it and enjoy it without hesitation. Why? Because your natural instincts cause you to be drawn to fruits and vegetables. These foods are your body's natural fuel source, and your brain is hardwired to know that.

Even Our Reproductive Anatomy
Says We Are Plant-Eaters

Human males have seminal vesicles—no other meat-eating animal has these important semen-collecting pouches as part of their reproductive anatomy. The seminal vesicles are paired sacculated pouches connected to the prostate, located at the base of the bladder. They collect fluids made by the prostate, which nourish and transport the sperm. In general, the volume of the ejaculate of a carnivore is very small compared to that of an herbivore. A human male's anatomy and function clearly say we are herbivores.

Take a Cue from Your Body

Our hands are made for gathering plants, not for ripping flesh. We cool ourselves by sweating, like most other plant-eating animals, rather than panting like carnivores. We drink our beverages by sipping, not by lapping like a dog or a cat. The exhaustive comparisons of our body traits with those of other animals prove that we have evolved over eons in an environment of plant-based foods. We were made to be plant-eaters, not meat-eaters. We are now paying the price for straying from our design with chronic illness and premature death.

Starchy plant foods like rice, potatoes, beans, and corn must comprise the bulk of our natural diet in order to provide sufficient calories for daily activities. To this centerpiece are added fresh fruits and vegetables. Meats, dairy products, and other delicacies must be reserved only for special occasions, if at all, in order to prevent diseases of malnutrition caused by overindulging in rich foods.

The Bortons Pass It On

The Bortons were anxious to share this information with their son and daughter. They knew both would have a hard time refuting the evidence I'd presented for the value of a plant-based diet. Most importantly, they looked forward to sharing recipes and delicious, nutritious meals with their kids and grandkids once everyone was in agreement about the best way to eat, the way our bodies tell us we are supposed to eat, for health and for life.

SUMMARY SHEET *from Dr. McDougall*

- *The ancestors of modern humans were believed to live almost exclusively on plant foods.*

- *Humans appear as only slightly remodeled chimpanzee-like apes who are near-vegetarians.*

- *Our teeth, jaws, and taste buds are designed to process plant foods, not meat.*

- *Our salivary and stomach juices digest plant parts efficiently.*

- *Our intestine is intricate and long for slow digestion of complex carbohydrates, while a carnivore, such as a cat, has a short, straight, tubular intestine for rapid elimination.*

- *Carnivores have livers with unlimited capacity to process cholesterol. Humans cannot rid themselves of the excess cholesterol they eat, because their liver is not designed for efficient cholesterol removal.*

- *Our metabolic and nutritional needs show that we are intended to live with nutrients that are available only in plants.*

- *Our instincts draw us to fruits and vegetables, while the thought of catching, killing, butchering, and/or eating animals for food is naturally repulsive.*

- *Even the male reproductive anatomy says we are supposed to be plant-eaters.*

- *We are now paying the price for straying from our natural design with chronic illness and premature death.*

CHAPTER 15

Shopping, Cooking, and Comfort Foods Galore

B y now you have discovered the exciting secret of the McDougall Program—it's in the starches! Why is this exciting? Because most people think of starches as "comfort foods," foods that just plain make you feel good. But many fear that eating an abundance of starches will cause them to become overweight. Not true. When you look around the world at the hundreds of millions of people living primarily on starches, like rice for Chinese and Japanese populations, do you see people characterized by obesity? Certainly not.

And here's more good news—not only does the McDougall way of eating allow you to eat those wonderful comfort foods, it also encourages eating as *much* of them as you want. In fact, the *more* you eat of the *right* things, the *healthier* and *thinner* you will become.

When I had shared this last bit of information with Louise and Larry, they were ecstatic. Louise, however, had a hard time believing she was really going to get thinner by eating all she wanted. "You mean even though we're going on a diet, it's not really a diet at all? And we're still going to lose weight? That just sounds too good to be true."

Larry added, "One of my all-time favorite 'comfort foods' is mashed potatoes. So you're telling me that since potatoes are a starch, I can eat all the mashed potatoes I want on your diet and *still* lose weight?"

"Yes, Larry," I reassured him, "you can have all the mashed potatoes you want, BUT . . ."

"Always a but," interjected Louise.

"But you won't prepare them with two sticks of butter and a pint of half-and-half like before. There's really no comfort in knowing you're clogging up your arteries and layering fat onto your body. However, by preparing your creamy potatoes with flavorful vegetable broth, salt, pepper, and chives, you'll be indulging in real comfort food—knowing you're being good to your body as well as to your taste buds."

"That sounds pretty good, Dr. McDougall. I think we can do that." Larry was actually anxious to run home and try this new way of preparing an old favorite.

It was shortly after this visit with the Bortons that my wife, Mary, sat down with Louise to talk about possible alternatives for her and Larry's favorite forbidden foods. Mary also gave Louise the following tips on shopping and cooking à la McDougall and provided her with lists of foods to have on hand so that she and Larry would be set for success in their journey back to health.

The McDougall Diet: Foods to Enjoy

- Whole grains and whole grain cereals, such as brown rice, barley, corn, millet, quinoa, oatmeal, bulgur wheat, and wheat berries.

- Whole grain products, such as pastas, bread, tortillas, cereals, and puffed grains.

- Squashes, including acorn, buttercup, butternut, pumpkin, summer squash, and zucchini.

- Roots and tubers, including potatoes, sweet potatoes, yams, carrots, beets, rutabagas, and turnips.

- Beans and other legumes, such as adzuki, black beans, garbanzo, lentils, kidney beans, navy beans, pinto beans, peas, split peas, and string beans.

- Leafy green vegetables, such as broccoli, cabbage, collard greens, kale, various kinds of lettuces, spinach, mustard greens, and watercress.

- Green, yellow, and red vegetables, such as celery, cauliflower, asparagus, and tomatoes.

- Fruits, such as apples, bananas, berries, grapefruit, melons, oranges, peaches, and pears. (Limit servings of fruit to two or three per day.)

There are an endless number of ways to prepare these healthful starch-based foods to make them truly delicious and satisfying. I recommend that people start out by eating a lot of the foods they ate while growing up. Therefore, if you were raised on potatoes, then use lots of different recipes for potatoes. Likewise, if rice is a familiar ingredient from your past, try a wide variety of rice recipes. Choose recipes that contain your favorite spices, making adjustments to your own personal taste as needed. Of course, when you become more adventurous, you'll want to try dishes with unfamiliar vegetables and spices. Pick one or two recipes at a time that look interesting and contain ingredients and spices you have enjoyed in other recipes. You'll have no problem finding about a dozen recipes to begin with so that you won't be eating the same thing all the time.

Foods Not Allowed

The following is a list of the foods that are not allowed on the McDougall Diet, with ideas for possible substitutions.

DON'T EAT	POSSIBLE SUBSTITUTES
Cow's milk (for cereal or cooking)	Soymilk, rice milk, fruit juice, water
Cow's milk (as beverage)	Water, juice, herbal tea, cereal beverages
Butter	None, or use vegetable spreads
Cheese	Plant-based cheeses, such as soy, rice, or nut (in small amounts)
Cottage cheese	Mashed silken tofu
Yogurt	Soy yogurt (in small amounts)
Sour cream	Tofu sour cream (in small amounts)

DON'T EAT	POSSIBLE SUBSTITUTES
Ice cream	Pure fruit sorbet, frozen juice bars; soy or rice "ice cream" (as a treat)
Eggs (in cooking)	Ener-G Egg Replacer
Eggs (for eating)	None, or scrambled tofu
Meat, poultry, fish	Starchy vegetables, whole grains, pastas, beans
Mayonnaise	Tofu mayonnaise (in small amounts)
Vegetable oils (for pans)	None; use nonstick or silicone pots and pans
Vegetable oils (in recipes)	None; omit oil or replace oil with water or other liquids
White rice (refined)	Whole grain brown rice, other whole grains
White flour (refined)	Whole grain flours
Refined and sugar-coated cereals	Any oil-free, whole grain hot or cold cereal
Chocolate	Carob powder, nonfat cocoa powder (in small amounts)
Coffee, decaffeinated coffee, and black tea	Caffeine-free herbal tea, cereal beverages, hot water with lemon
Colas and other soft drinks	Mineral water or seltzer (flavored or plain)

As you try various new dishes, you will undoubtedly stumble upon family favorites. When you do, please remember that it's OK to enjoy the same favorite dishes again and again. Given the health-promoting nature of the foods you will be consuming, it will be fine to eat the same thing for breakfast, lunch, and dinner. Consider populations following a typical Asian diet—they eat rice and vegetables three times a day and are virtually free of coronary heart disease, diabetes, obesity, gallstones, constipation, and colon cancer!

Healthful Shopping Habits

After choosing the meals you'd like to enjoy, make a shopping list based on the week's menu. You'll then want to locate a store that sells healthful grains, vegetables, beans, fruits, snacks, condiments, and supplies. Have fun—this is an exciting time! You are choosing tasty new foods to fill your pantry and refrigerator, and because these are healthful foods, you'll be eating to your heart's content. Now that's exciting!

Fortunately, finding food stores that meet the standards of health-conscious eaters is becoming easier. Natural food stores have been expanding to the size of supermarkets during the last two decades. They sell everything from dog food to toilet paper (recycled, of course). The success of these natural food stores has forced other supermarkets to meet consumers' demands for more healthful products. Also, increased sales volume has brought down the cost of healthful foods in both traditional supermarkets and natural food markets.

Reading labels is the key to effective food shopping. Ingredients are supposed to be listed in descending order of amounts contained in the package. However, these labels can be deceptive. Sometimes simple sugars (such as sucrose, corn syrup, fructose, and fruit concentrate) are listed individually in order to move "sugar" from the first and primary ingredient to a position farther down the list. Since you will be avoiding fats, it is important to understand that manufacturers have also found ways of hiding fats in ingredient lists by calling them "monoglycerides" or "diglycerides." You might recognize "triglyceride" as being a complex fat (in your bloodstream), but may fail to recognize the mono- and di- forms, or you may think they are additives unrelated to fats. Lecithin is another fat you may not recognize as such. Products with oils listed as ingredients should be avoided, as well as those containing dairy products, which are often concealed on the ingredient list as whey, casein, milk solids, and lactose.

Keep an assortment of healthful ingredients readily available in the kitchen so that sudden hunger pangs are quelled by good foods rather than by a trip to the nearest fast food joint. This means planning ahead. In our home we always make sure that we have a well-stocked pantry and refrigerator so that we can whip up a family favorite at a moment's notice without making a special trip to the supermarket. These are some of the ingredients we always have on hand so that we can prepare a wide variety of quick and easy meals. Items followed by an asterisk (*) are made of simple sugars or flours and should be reduced or eliminated for more effective weight loss and control of triglycerides. Items followed by two asterisks (**) tend to be high in sodium.

The Well-Stocked Pantry

PANTRY SHELF STAPLES

Apple juice *

Applesauce *

Baking powder (aluminum-free) **

Baking soda **

Barbecue sauce (oil-free) **

Beans, canned (rinse before using)

Chiles, canned green **

Beans, dried (pinto beans, Great Northern beans, garbanzos, black beans, etc.)

Beans, fat-free refried, canned **

Coffee substitutes (Teeccino, Roma, etc.)

Cold cereals (check for fats and sodium)

Cornstarch

Dip and dressing mixes (Simply Organic, Hain, Bearitos) **

Dr. McDougall's Right Foods Smart Cups

Ener-G Egg Replacer

Flour, whole wheat or unbleached white *

Fruit, dried (prunes, raisins, currants, figs, dates, apricots, etc.) *

Herbal teas

Honey * or Agave Nectar *

Hot sauce (Tabasco, hot chili sauce, etc.) **

Kabuli pizza crust * (to order, call Dallas Gourmet Bakery at 972-247-9835)

Ketchup **

Maple syrup (pure) *

Mayonnaise, fat-free (Nasoya Nayonaise) **

Molasses *

Mustard

Oats, rolled (oatmeal) and steel-cut

Olives, ripe (high fat) **

Pasta, wheat or rice (high fat)

Pasta sauce (check for fat and sodium)

Peanut butter (only peanuts and salt) * **

Pimiento pieces **

Salad dressings, fat-free (Honey Mustard, Italian, French) **

Salsa **

Soymilk or rice milk, in aseptic cartons

Soy sauce, low-sodium

Sugar, brown or Sucanat *

Taco seasoning mix (Bearitos)

Tahini (high fat)

Tomatoes, chopped canned (including seasoned) **

Tomato juice or V-8 juice **

Tomato sauce and paste **

Vegetable broth * **

Vegetables, canned (artichokes, roasted red peppers, beets, pumpkin) **

Vinegar (rice, wine, balsamic)

Whole grains (brown rice, barley, oats, and others, as desired)

Wonderslim Cocoa Powder *

Wonderslim Fat Replacer *

Worcestershire sauce, vegetarian **

FRESH FOODS FOR YOUR PANTRY

Bread, low-fat, low-sodium (from a local bakery, or 100% whole grain flours) *

Garlic

Onions

Potatoes

Tomatoes

The Well-Stocked Refrigerator

PACKAGED ITEMS

Garlic, bottled minced

Ginger, bottled minced

Jelly or jam *

Lemon juice

Lime juice

Miso **

Salsa (store-bought or homemade) **

Soy or rice cheese, (high fat) **

Soymilk or rice milk (fresh)

Tofu, silken and water-packed (high fat)

FRESH VEGETABLES

Avocado (high fat)

Bell peppers, green or red

Broccoli (optional)

Carrots

Cauliflower (optional)

Celery

Cilantro (optional)

Lettuce

Mushrooms

Onions, green

Parsley (optional)

Snow peas

Spinach (optional)

Sprouts (optional)

Squash, summer or winter
   (optional)

FRESH FRUIT *

Apples

Bananas

Grapes

Oranges, tangerines or
    grapefruit

Seasonal fruit

The Well-Stocked Freezer

Buns, whole wheat *

Burgers, meat-free, soy-free * **

Potatoes, hash-brown

Sorbet *

Tortillas, corn (made only with corn, water, and lime)

Tortillas, whole wheat *

Vegetables, plain (corn, peas, spinach, etc.)

The Well-Stocked Seasoning Cabinet

Allspice

Basil

Bay leaf

Cayenne

Celery Seed

Chili powder

Cinnamon

Cloves

Coriander

Crushed red pepper

Cumin, ground

Curry powder

Dill seed

Dill weed

Dry mustard

Garlic powder

Marjoram

Nutmeg

Onion powder

Oregano

Paprika

Parsley flakes

Pepper

Rosemary

Sage

Salt

Tarragon

Thyme

Turmeric

Vanilla extract

Snack Foods (use sparingly) **

Black bean dip, fat-free	Popcorn
Corn cakes (Corn Thins)	Pretzels *
Crackers, fat-free rice or wheat *	Rice cakes
Hummus, fat-free	Tortilla chips, baked

Cookware

(Avoid cookware that allows aluminum to touch your foods)

Baking dishes, various sizes

Baking sheets, nonstick

Cake pans, various sizes (silicone, or use parchment paper)

Casserole dishes, various sizes, with covers

Colanders and strainers, various sizes

Griddle, nonstick

Pasta pot, with insert

Saucepans, various sizes

Skillet, nonstick large

Slow cooker

Soup pot, large

Loaf pans (silicone, or use parchment paper)

Muffin cups (silicone)

Pressure cooker (optional)

Rice cooker (optional, but you'll be glad you have it!)

Teakettle

Tools

Cutting board	Ladle
Fork, large	Spatula
Knives (a good-quality chef's knife is very important!)	Spoon, slotted
	Spoons, wooden, various sizes

Where to Find Recipes

Hundreds of delicious recipes are available on the McDougall Web site at www.drmcdougall.com and in all of the McDougall books. I especially recommend the *McDougall Quick and Easy Cookbook*.

Seasoning Foods

So much of a food's flavor depends on the way it is prepared and on the seasonings, sauces, and dressings used to enhance the flavor. Use the delicious recipes in the many McDougall cookbooks as guidelines, but feel free to experiment. Have fun substituting your own favorite spices, adjust the amount of recommended seasonings to fit your own taste, or even combine recipes if you wish!

The two most popular seasonings are salt and sugar—and for a very good reason: the tip of the tongue is covered with taste buds that are sensitive to and satisfied by the flavors of salt and sugar. Nature designed us to desire sweet-tasting carbohydrates, because these foods are the richest in nutrition and energy. In order to most fully enjoy salt and sugar—and avoid damaging your health from overuse—sprinkle these two condiments on the surface of food, where your tongue can easily contact them.

Browning Vegetables Without Oil

Browned onions have an excellent flavor and can be used alone or mixed with other vegetables to make a mouth-watering dish. To achieve the color of browning, as well as to flavor your foods, place 1 1/2 cups of chopped onions in a large nonstick skillet with 1 cup of water or vegetable broth. Cook over medium heat, stirring occasionally, until the liquid evaporates and the onions begin to stick to the bottom of the pan. Continue to stir for one minute, then add another 1/2 cup of water or broth, loosening the browned bits from the bottom of the pan. Cook until the liquid evaporates again. Repeat this procedure one or two more times until the onions are as browned as you'd like. You can also use this technique to brown carrots, green peppers, garlic, potatoes, shallots, zucchini, and many other vegetables, alone or in interesting combinations.

Baking Without Oil

Eliminating oil in baking is a real challenge, because oil keeps baked goods moist and soft. Replace the oil called for in the recipe with half the amount of another moist food, such as applesauce, mashed bananas, mashed potatoes, mashed pumpkin, tomato sauce, soft silken tofu, or soy yogurt (keep in mind that tofu and soy yogurt are high-fat foods). There are several fat replacers on the market, for example, Wonderslim Fat and Egg Replacer and Sunsweet Lighter Bake.

Cakes and muffins made without oil usually come out a little heavier. For a lighter texture, use carbonated water instead of tap water in baking recipes. Be sure to test cakes and muffins at the end of the baking time by inserting a toothpick or a cake tester in the center to see if it comes out clean. Sometimes oil-free cakes and muffins may need to bake longer than the directions advise, depending on the weather or the altitude at which you live.

Sautéing Without Oil

To sauté implies the use of butter or oil, but when cooking the McDougall way, oil is eliminated. Instead, we use other liquids to provide taste without the health hazards. Surprisingly, plain water makes an excellent sautéing liquid. It prevents foods from sticking to the pan and still allows vegetables to brown and cook. For additional flavor, try sautéing in one of the following:

Soy sauce (tamari)

Vegetable broth

Red or white wine (alcoholic or nonalcoholic)

Sherry (alcoholic or nonalcoholic)

Rice vinegar or balsamic vinegar

Tomato juice

Lemon or lime juice

Salsa

Worcestershire sauce

For even more taste, add herbs and/or spices (such as ginger, dry mustard, or garlic) to the above liquids.

Dinner with the Bortons

Six months after Louise's cooking class with my wife, Mary, the Bortons invited us to their home for dinner. When the evening arrived, we were greeted at the door by savory aromas and also by a trim, healthy couple who looked far different from the Larry and Louise who had walked into my office over a year and a half before.

Larry said, "Dr. McDougall, I told you when we first met that if you could help us get healthy, we'd have you over for dinner to celebrate. Well, obviously we're down a few sizes, but the best thing is we have our lives back."

The Bortons welcomed Mary and me into their home, where pictures of grandkids covered every available wall—one a recent photo of Larry rock climbing with his grandson. As we sat down at the dinner table, Louise said, "I know back when we first met we promised prime rib and all the trimmings, with cheesecake for dessert, but I'm sure you'll be delighted to see the menu's changed a little. Instead we're having Broccoli Bisque, Quinoa Garden Salad, and Shepherd's Pie, and we'll finish it off with my favorite dessert, Chocolate Decadence Pudding."

Larry related that once they had stocked their kitchen with healthful foods, they found it easier to eat well. Learning to substitute healthful ingredients for unhealthful ones enabled Louise to make some of their favorite meals, often simply by removing animal fats and oils from the sauces.

"I thought eating like this all the time would be boring," Louise admitted. "It's actually been like a culinary adventure—trying lots of new recipes, experimenting with ingredients. We definitely do *not* feel deprived eating things like oatmeal, bean burritos, minestrone soup, chili, and lasagne. How could it be boring when we have literally hundreds of McDougall recipes to choose from?"

"Our lives are so much easier now." Larry explained. "Before, we suffered from constant aches and pains and were always worried

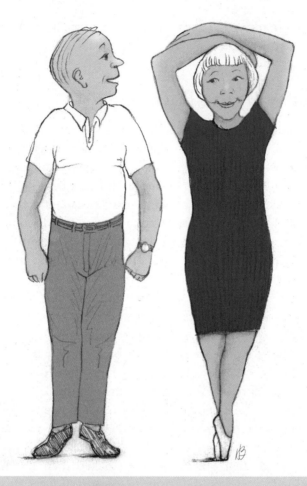

Larry and Louise are now enjoying an easy life—free from the burdens of being overweight, in pain, and living with impaired bodily functions.

about our health. We had to take all kinds of medications, and waiting around in doctor's offices was no fun either."

Louise continued, "And I had to shop in the plus-size section of the clothing store—now *that* was difficult."

"We look at things so differently now. I was watching my brother wolf down a pepperoni pizza the other day and thought to myself, it is no mystery why he is so fat and has to take cholesterol, blood pressure, diabetes, and antacid pills. I am amazed that so many people, even doctors, fail to see the obvious. Thank you, Dr. McDougall, for opening our eyes," Larry said.

"No, thank you, Larry and Louise, for giving me the opportunity to provide the most rewarding of all services—and that is to help others. I'm the luckiest doctor in the world—my patients get healthier," I said to them fondly before sitting down to our delicious dinner. "And I hope all of our future meetings are casual, like this, and not as a doctor and a patient. Congratulations! You have escaped from the medical and pharmaceutical businesses by becoming healthy."

Like the Bortons, you will find that with over 2,200 recipes published in the McDougall books and newsletters, discovering new favorites will be an enjoyable adventure. You will eventually come up with some of your very own unique recipes. When you do, we'd love for you to share them with us by writing to us at office@drmcdougall.com.

I am confident that as you begin to fill your body with flavorful, healthful foods, you will be well on your way to looking and feeling better than you ever imagined possible. As Louise said, eating the foods that are good for you does not have to be boring. And as Larry said, this is undoubtedly the easy way to live. By following our tips and guidelines, and taking advantage of the other McDougall resources, like Larry and Louise you will find yourself embarking on a "culinary adventure," and most importantly—taking back your health and your life.

Delicious McDougall recipes are found here. . .

WEBSITE

www.drmcdougall.com

BOOKS

The McDougall Quick & Easy Cookbook

The New McDougall Cookbook

The McDougall Program—12 Days to Dynamic Health

The McDougall Program for Maximum Weight Loss

Other Books by John A. McDougall, MD. . .

McDougall's Medicine: A Challenging Second Opinion

The McDougall Program for Women

The McDougall Program for a Healthy Heart

DVD SETS

Dr. McDougall's Total Health Solution for the 21st Century

McDougall's Medicine: Fighting the Big Fat Lies with Fad-Free Truth

Notes

The nutritional values used throughout this book are obtained from the following source:

Jean A. Pennington, Anna De Planter Bowes, and Helen Nichols Church, *Bowes & Church's food values of portions commonly used* 17th edition (Philadelphia and New York: Lippincott, 1998).

CHAPTER 2

One-quarter of medical schools require training in the medical nutrition sciences:

R. F. Kushner et al., "Implementing Nutrition into the Medical Curriculum: A User's Guide, *Am J Clin Nutr* 52, no. 2 (August 1990): 401–03;

D. C. Heimburger, V. A. Stallings, and L. Routzahn, "Survey of Clinical Nutrition Training Programs for Physicians," *Am J Clin Nutr* 68, no. 6 (December 1998): 1174–79.

Worldwide, the trimmest, healthiest, most youthful people live on plant-based, high-carbohydrate diets:

P. T. James, "Obesity: The Worldwide Epidemic," *Clin Dermatol* 22, no. 4 (July–August 2004): 276–80;

J. H. Weisburger, "Eat to Live, Not Live to Eat," *Nutrition* 16, no. 9 (September 2000): 767–73.

Migration and change of diet means more obesity and Western disease:

M. S. Goel et al., "Obesity Among US Immigrant Subgroups by Duration of Residence, *JAMA* 292, no. 23 (December 2004): 2860–67;

M. S. Kaplan et al., "The Association Between Length of Residence and Obesity among Hispanic Immigrants," *Am J Prev Med* 27, no. 4 (November 2004): 323–26.

Wealth from industrialization means more rich foods and disease;

> K. G. Alberti, P. Zimmet, J. Shaw, and IDF Epidemiology Task Force Consensus Group, "The Metabolic Syndrome—A New Worldwide Definition," *Lancet* 366, no. 9491 (September 2005): 1059–62.

CHAPTER 3

Between 50 and 60 percent of the population suffer from chronic halitosis:

> J. P. Meningaud et al., "Halitosis in 1999," *Rev Stomatol Chir Maxillofac* 100, no. 5 (October 1999): 240–44.

A woman's odor heightens her attractiveness to a man:

> D. Singh and P. M. Bronstad, "Female Body Odour Is a Potential Cue to Ovulation," *Proc Biol Sci* 268, no. 1469 (April 2001): 797–801.

Women prefer the body odor of dominant men:

> J. Havlicek, S. C. Roberts, and J. Flegr, *Biol. Lett* doi 10, 1098/rsbl (2005).

Food determines body odor:

> J. H. Cummings, "Fermentation in the Human Large Intestine: Evidence and Implications for Health," *Lancet* 1, no. 8335 (May 1983): 1206–09;

> M. Smith, L. G. Smith, and B. Levinson, "The Use of Smell in Differential Diagnosis," *Lancet* 2, no. 8313 (December 1982): 1452–53.

Natural adaptations to odors occur within the nervous system:

> P. Dalton, "Psychophysical and Behavioral Characteristics of Olfactory Adaptation," *Chem Senses* 25, no. 4 (August 2000): 487–92.

Most common cause of offensive breath odor is sulfur:

> S. Awano et al., "The Assessment of Methyl Mercaptan: An Important Clinical Marker for the Diagnosis of Oral Malodor," *J Dent* 32, no. 7 (September 2004): 555–59.

Brushing the teeth and ingestion of breath tablets fail:

> F. L. Suarez et al., "Morning Breath Odor: Influence of Treatments on Sulfur Gases," *J Dent Res* 79, no. 10 (October 2000): 1773–77.

Zinc mouthwashes directly oxidize gaseous sulfur:

> K. Yaegaki and J. M. Coil, "Examination, Classification, and Treatment of Halitosis: Clinical Perspectives," *J Can Dent Assoc* 66 (2000): 257–61.

Sulfur gases cause inflammation, known as periodontitis:

> P. A. Ratcliff and P. W. Johnson, "The Relationship Between Oral Malodor, Gingivitis, and Periodontitis," *J Periodontol* 70, no. 5 (May 1999): 485–89.

Periodontal disease is associated with heart disease:

> J. Katz, "Inflammation, Periodontitis, and Coronary Heart Disease," *Lancet*, 2001, 358:303.

Sulfur gases cause ulcerative colitis:

> W. Babidge, S. Millard, and W. Roediger, "Sulfides Impair Short Chain Fatty Acid Beta-Oxidation at Acyl-CoA Dehydrogenase Level in Colonocytes: Implications for Ulcerative Colitis," *Mol Cell Biochem* 181, no. 1–2 (April 1998): 117–24.

Higher levels of homocysteine mean more diseases:

> M. P. Mattson and F. Haberman, "Folate and Homocysteine Metabolism: Therapeutic Targets in Cardiovascular and Neurodegenerative Disorders," *Curr Med Chem* 10, no. 19 (October 2003): 1923–29.

CHAPTER 4

Fifty-six percent of people in Western countries report indigestion:

> T. D. Bolin, "Heartburn: Community Perceptions," *J Gastroenterol Hepatol* 15, no. 1 (January 2000): 35–39.

Indigestion is worse than heart failure, symptomatic heart disease, diabetes, and hypertension:

> D. A. Revicki, "The Impact of Gastroesophageal Reflux Disease on Health-Related Quality of Life," *Am J Med* 104, no. 3 (March 1998): 252–58;

> H. Glise, "Quality of Life Assessments in the Evaluation of Gastroesophageal Reflux and Peptic Ulcer Disease Before, During and After Treatment," *Scand J Gastroenterol* Suppl 208 (1995): 133–35.

Sales of antacids including, Prilosec and Prevacid:

> National Institute for Health Care Management, "Prescription Drug Expenditures in the Year 2001: Another Year of Escalating Costs" (revised May 6, 2002) http://www. nihcm.org/spending2001.pdf.

Well-respected researcher from Yale University believes 90 percent of GERD from constipation:

> S. J. Sontag, "Defining GERD," *Yale J Biol Med* 72, no. 2–3 (March–June 1999): 69–80.

Best diet for losing weight permanently is high carbohydrate:

> A. Astrup et al., "Low-fat Diets and Energy Balance: How Does the Evidence Stand in 2002?" *Proc Nutr Soc* 61, no. 2 (May 2002): 299–309.

Avoid consumption of dairy products, which cause constipation by paralyzing the muscles of the bowels:

> G. Iacono, "Intolerance of Cow's Milk and Chronic Constipation in Children," *N Engl J Med* 339, no. 16 (October 1998): 1100–04.

Dietary fiber is a cure for constipation:

W. Scheppach, "Beneficial Health Effects of Low-digestible Carbohydrate Consumption," *Br J Nutr* 85, Suppl 1 (March 2001): S23–30.

Thirty years ago a high-fat diet was recognized as a cause of acidity, heartburn, and belching:

P. Childs, "Dietary fat, Dyspepsia, Diarrhoea, and Diabetes," *Br J Surg* 59 (1972): 669–95.

University of Virginia Health Sciences Center confirmed that fat causes heartburn:

R. H. Holloway, "Effect of Intraduodenal Fat on Lower Oesophageal Sphincter Function and Gastro-oesophageal Reflux," *Gut* 40, no. 4 (April 1997): 449–53.

Heartburn becomes progressively worse three hours after a meal high in fat:

D. Becker, "A Comparison of High and Low Fat Meals on Postprandial Esophageal Acid Exposure," *Am J Gastroenterol* 84, no. 7 (July 1989): 782–86.

Large fatty meals, which overdistend the stomach, are a major cause of heartburn:

R. H. Holloway, "Gastric Distention: A Mechanism for Postprandial Gastroesophageal Reflux," *Gastroenterology* 89, no. 4 (October 1985): 779–84.

Coffee and decaf cause indigestion and reflux:

G. Van Deventer, "Lower Esophageal Sphincter Pressure, Acid Secretion, and Blood Gastrin After Coffee Consumption," *Dig Dis Sci* 37, no. 4 (April 1992): 558–69;

B. Wendl, "Effect of Decaffeination of Coffee or Tea on Gastro-oesophageal Reflux," *Aliment Pharmacol Ther* 8, no. 3 (June 1994): 283–87;

C. Pehl, "The Effect of Decaffeination of Coffee on Gastro-oesophageal Reflux in Patients with Reflux Disease," *Aliment Pharmacol Ther* 11, no. 3 (June 1997): 483–86;

S. Cohen, "Gastric Acid Secretion and Lower-Esophageal-Sphincter Pressure in Response to Coffee and Caffeine," *N Engl J Med* 293, no. 18 (October 1975): 897–99.

No increase in the risk of stomach or duodenal ulcers with coffee drinkers:

G. H. Elta, "Comparison of Coffee Intake and Coffee-Induced Symptoms in Patients with Duodenal Ulcer, Nonulcer Dyspepsia, and Normal Controls," *Am J Gastroenterol* 85, no. 10 (October 1990): 1339–42.

Cigarette smoking and alcohol can compromise LES function and cause indigestion:

C. F. Smit, "Effect of Cigarette Smoking on Gastropharyngeal and Gastroesophageal Reflux," *Ann Otol Rhinol Laryngol* 110, no. 2 (February 2001): 190–93;

D. Weinberg, "The Diagnosis and Management of Gastroesophageal Reflux Disease," *Med Clin North Am* 80, no. 2 (March 1996): 411–29;

W. Hogan, "Ethanol-Induced Acute Esophageal Motor Dysfunction," *J Appl Physiol* 32, no. 6 (June 1972): 755–60.

Wine and beer cause more indigestion than distilled beverages:

S. Teyssen, "Maleic Acid and Succinic Acid in Fermented Alcoholic Beverages are the Stimulants of Gastric Acid Secretion," *J Clin Invest* 103, no. 5 (March 1999): 707–13.

Onions cause indigestion and reflux:

M. L. Allen, "The Effect of Raw Onions on Acid Reflux and Reflux Symptoms," *Am J Gastroenterol* 85, no. 4 (April 1990): 377–80.

Chocolate lowers LES pressure:

D. Murphy, "Chocolate and Heartburn: Evidence of Increased Esophageal Acid Exposure after Chocolate Ingestion," *Am J Gastroenterol* 83, no. 6 (June 1988): 633–36;

J. Babka, "On the Genesis of Heartburn: The Effects of Specific Foods on the Lower Esophageal Sphincter," *Am J Dig Dis* 18, no. 5 (May 1973): 391–97.

Approximately 40 percent of people surveyed had symptoms of heartburn after chocolate:

O. Nebel, "Symptomatic gastroesophageal reflux: incidence and precipitating factors," *Am J Dig Dis* 21 (1976): 953–56.

Citrus fruits, tomatoes, and spicy foods have a direct irritating effect:

S. Price, "Food Sensitivity in Reflux Esophagitis," *Am J Gastroenterol* 75 (1978): 240–43;

J. P. Cranley, "Abnormal Lower Esophageal Sphincter Pressure Responses in Patients with Orange Juice-Induced Heartburn," *Am J Gastroenterol* 81, no. 2 (February 1986): 104–06.

Individuals with dental erosions have GERD:

P. Schroeder, "Dental Erosion and Acid Reflux Disease," *Ann Intrn Med* 122 (1995): 809–15;

J. N. Groen and A. J. Smout, "Supra-oesophageal Manifestations of Gastro-oesophageal Reflux Disease," *Eur J Gastroenterol Hepatol* 15, no. 12 (December 2003): 1339–50.

Acid refluxed up into the back of the throat causes asthma:

W. Simpson, "Gastroesophageal Reflux Risease and Asthma: Diagnosis and Management," *Arch Intrn Med* 155 (1995): 798–803;

B. Gopal, P. Singhal, and S. N. Gaur, "Gastroesophageal Reflux Disease in Bronchial Asthma and the Response to Omeprazole," *Asian Pac J Allergy Immunol* 23, no. 1 (March 2005): 29–34.

Raising the head of the bed by four to six inches relieves asthma:

W. Hogan, "Medical Treatment of Supraesophageal Complications of Gastroesophageal Reflux Disease," *Am J Med* 111, Suppl 8A (December 2001): 197S–201S.

Reflux causes otitis media in children:

A. Tasker et al., "Reflux of Gastric Juice and Glue Ear in Children," *Lancet* 359, no. 9305 (February 2002): 493.

Fast food restaurants and indigestion:

S. Rodriguez, "Meal Type Affects Heartburn Severity," *Dig Dis Sci* 43, no. 3 (March 1998): 485–90.

Proton pump inhibitors may cause stomach cancer with long-term use:

D. C. Farrow, "Gastroesophageal Reflux Disease: Use of H2 Receptor Antagonists and Risk of Esophageal and Gastric Cancer," *Cancer Causes Control* 11, no. 3 (March 2000): 231–38.

CHAPTER 5

One study, eight men and four women were fed one ounce of freshly ground jalapeño chiles:

D. Graham, "Spicy Food and the Stomach: Evaluation by Videoendoscopy," *JAMA* 260 (1988): 3473–75.

No difference in inflammation and healing with heavy spice:

K. Tyagi, "Gastric Mucosal Morphology in Tropics and Influence of Spices, Tea, and Smoking," *Nutr Metab* 17 (1974): 129–35;

N. Kumar, "Do Chilies Influence Healing of Duodenal Ulcer?" *BMJ* 288 (1984): 1803–04.

In rats, capsaicin protects from damage caused by alcohol or aspirin:

P. Holzer, "Intragastric Capsaicin Protects Against Aspirin-Induced Lesion Formation and Bleeding in Rat Gastric Mucosa," *Gastroenterlogy* 96, no. 6 (June 1989): 1425–33;

P. Holzer, "Stimulation of Afferant Nerve Endings by Intragastric Capsaicin Protects Against Ethanol-Induced Damage of Gastric Mucosa," *Neuroscience* 27 (1988): 981–87.

Sippy Diet does not heal ulcers and causes heart disease:

> R. Briggs, "Myocardial Infarction in Patients Treated with Sippy and Other High-Milk Diets: An Autopsy Study of Fifteen Hospitals in the USA and Great Britain," *Circulation* 21 (1960): 538.

Over eighty years ago scientists reported that milk was a strong acid-producing stimulant and milk and egg was worse:

> B. Crohn, *Am J Med Sci* 59 (1920): 70.

In the mid 1970s, researchers concluded, "Because milk contains both protein and calcium . . .":

> A. F. Ippoliti, "The Effect of Various Forms of Milk on Gastric-Acid Secretion: Studies in Patients with Duodenal Ulcer and Normal Subjects," *Ann Intern Med* 84, no. 3 (March 1976): 286–89.

Animal protein is more acid-producing than plant protein:

> F. P. Brooks, "Effect of Diet on Gastric Secretion," *Am J Clin Nutr* 42, Suppl 5 (November 1985): 1006–19.

Acid secretion 30–40 percent less with soy protein than with beef protein:

> K. E. McArthur, "Soy Protein Meals Stimulate Less Gastric Acid Secretion and Gastrin Release than Beef Meals," *Gastroenterology* 95, no. 4 (October 1988): 920–26.

Ulcers more common with milk, meat, and bread, and also total fat:

> S. Elmstahl, "Fermented Milk Products are Associated to Ulcer Diseases: Results from a Cross-Sectional Population Study," *Eur J Clin Nutr* 52 (1998): 668–74

Maleic and succinic acid from beer and wine during are the acid producing:

> S. Teyssen, "Maleic Acid and Succinic Acid in Fermented Alcoholic Beverages are the Stimulants of Gastric Acid Secretion," *J Clin Invest* 103, no. 5 (March 1999): 707–13.

About 15 percent of people who frequently take NSAIDs have gastric or duodenal ulcer.

> E. N. Larkai, "Gastroduodenal Mucosa and Dyspeptic Symptoms in Arthritic Patients during Chronic Nonsteroidal Anti-inflammatory Drug Use," *Am J Gastroenterol* 82, no. 11 (November 1987): 1153–58.

COX-2 inhibitor NSAIDs increase the chances of heart attack:

> S. R. Maxwell and D. J. Webb, "COX-2 Selective Inhibitors: Important Lessons Learned," *Lancet* 365, no. 9458 (February 2005): 449–51.

H. pylori in the stomachs of 70–90 percent of people in developing countries:

> B. Dunn, "Helicobacter pylori," Clin Microbiol Rev 10, no. 4 (October 1997): 720–41.

H. pylori is probably an "innocent bystander" for most patients:

>   H. Clearfield, "*Helicobacter pylori*: Aggressor or Innocent Bystander?"
>   *Med Clin North Am* 75, no. 4 (July 1991): 815–29;

>   P. Suadicani, "Genetic and Life-style Determinants of Peptic Ulcer: A
>   Study of 3387 Men Aged 54 to 74 years; The Copenhagen Male
>   Study," *Scand J Gastroenterol* 34, no. 1 (January 1999): 12–27.

NSAIDs and H. pylori are sixty-one times more likely to develop ulcers:

>   R. Pounder, "*Helicobacter pylori* and NSAIDs: The End of the Debate?"
>   *Lancet* 358 (2002): 3–4.

Fruits and vegetables and of vitamin C, appears to protect against infection
with H. pylori:

>   L. M. Brown, "*Helicobacter pylori*: Epidemiology and Routes of Trans-
>   mission," *Epidemiol Rev* 22, no. 2 (2000): 283–97;

>   G. Misciagna, "Diet and Duodenal Ulcer," *Dig Liver Dis* 32, no. 6
>   (August–September 2000): 468–72.

Garlic, thyme, and East African herbal plants, inhibit the growth of
H. pylori:

>   G. B. Mahady, "Allixin, a Phytoalexin from Garlic, Inhibits the Growth
>   of *Helicobacter pylori* in Vitro," *Am J Gastroenterol* 96, no. 12
>   (December 2001): 3454–55;

>   G. Sivan, "*Helicobacter pylori*: In Vitro Susceptibility to Garlic (Allium
>   sativum) Extract," *Nutr Cancer* 27 (1997): 118–21;

>   M. Tabak et al., "*In vitro* Inhibition of *Helicobacter pylori* by Extracts of
>   Thyme," *J. Appl. Microbiol* 80 (1996): 667–72;

>   W. Fabry, P. Okemo, and R. Ansborg, "Activity of East African Medici-
>   nal Plants Against *Helicobacter pylori*," *Chemotherapy* 42 (1996):
>   315–17.

Treatment of H. pylori with triple therapy:

>   P. Bytzer and C. O'Morain, "Treatment of *Helicobacter pylori*," *Helicobac-
>   ter* 10, Suppl 1 (2005): 40–46.

Triple therapy rarely relieves common indigestion:

>   P. Moayyedi et al., "Eradication of Helicobacter pylori for Non-ulcer
>   Dyspepsia," Cochrane Database Syst Rev, January 2005, no.
>   1:CD002096.

Broccoli and inhibition of H. pylori and ulcer treatment:

>   M. V. Galan, A. A. Kishan, and A. L. Silverman, "Oral Broccoli Sprouts
>   for the Treatment of *Helicobacter pylori* Infection: A Preliminary
>   Report," *Dig Dis Sci* 49, no. 7–9, (August 2004): 1088–90.

Cabbage juice to treat ulcers:

> R. Doll and F. Pygott, "Clinical Trial of Robaden and of Cabbage Juice in the Treatment of Gastric Ulcer," *Lancet* 267, no. 6850 (December 1954): 1200–04.

CHAPTER 6

Statistics on gallbladder disease:

> M. Tseng, "Dietary Intake and Gallbladder Disease: A Review," *Public Health Nutr* 2, no. 2 (June 1999): 161–72;

> J. E. Everhart, "Prevalence and Ethnic Differences in Gallbladder Disease in the United States," *Gastroenterology* 117, no. 3 (September 1999): 632–39;

> G. D. Friedman, "Natural History of Asymptomatic and Symptomatic Gallstones," *Am J Surg* 165, no. 4 (April 1993): 399–404.

Estrogen, body weight, cholesterol, and aging play roles in gallstone formation:

> S. Strasberg, "The Pathogenesis of Cholesterol Gallstones a Review, *J Gastrointest Surg* 2, no. 2 (March–April 1998): 109–25.

Supersaturation of the bile with cholesterol is the key to gallstone formation:

> P. Portincasa et al., "Modulation of Cholesterol Crystallization in Bile: Implications for Non-surgical Treatment of Cholesterol Gallstone Disease," *Curr Drug Targets Immune Endocr Metabol Disord* 5, no. 2 (June 2005): 177–84.

Dietary fat encourages gallstone formation:

> A. Cuevas et al., "Diet as a Risk Factor for Cholesterol Gallstone Disease," *J Am Coll Nutr* 23, no. 3 (June 2004): 187–96.

Dietary fiber reduces the risk of gallstones:

> C. J. Tsai et al., "Long-term Intake of Dietary Fiber and Decreased Risk of Cholecystectomy in Women," *Am J Gastroenterol* 99, no. 7 (July 2004): 1364–70;

> R. Dowling, Review. Pathogenesis of Gallstones," *Aliment Pharmacol Ther* 14, Suppl 2 (May 2000): 39–47.

No other animal besides the human is known to spontaneously develop cholesterol gallstones:

> K. C. Hayes, A. Livingston, and E. A. Trautwein, "Dietary Impact on Biliary Lipids and Gallstones," *Annu Rev Nutr*, 1992, no. 12:299–326.

Prevalence of gallstones worldwide:

> W. Kratzer, R. A. Mason, and V. Kachele, "Prevalence of Gallstones in Sonographic Surveys Worldwide," *J Clin Ultrasound* 27, no. 1 (January 1999): 1–7;

E. A. Shaffer, "Epidemiology and Risk Factors for Gallstone Disease: Has the Paradigm Changed in the 21st Century?" *Curr Gastroenterol Rep* 7, no. 2 (May 2005): 132–40.

Gallstones and American Indians:

J. E. Everhart et al., "Prevalence of Gallbladder Disease in American Indian Populations: Findings from the Strong Heart Study," *Hepatology* 35, no. 6 (June 2002): 1507–12;

M. Acalovschi, "Cholesterol Gallstones: From Epidemiology to Prevention," *Postgrad Med J* 77, no. 906 (April 2001): 221–29.

Gallstones once rare in Japan;

M. Nagase et al., "Present Features of Gallstones in Japan: A Collective Review of 2,144 Cases," *Am J Surg* 135, no. 6 (June 1978): 788–90.

Vegetarians rarely have gallbladder disease:

F. Pixley, "Effect of Vegetarianism on Development of Gall Stones in Women," *Br Med J (Clin Res Ed)* 291, no. 6487 (July 1985):11–12;

W. Kratzer, "Gallstone Prevalence in Relation to Smoking, Alcohol, Coffee Consumption, and Nutrition," The Ulm Gallstone Study, *Scand J Gastroenterol* 32, no. 9 (September 1997): 953–58;

P. Nair and J. F. Mayberry, "Vegetarianism, Dietary Fibre and Gastrointestinal Disease," *Dig Dis* 12, no. 3 (May–June 1994): 177–85.

Weight loss and gallstones:

S. Erlinger, "Gallstones in Obesity and Weight Loss," *Eur J Gastroenterol Hepatol* 12, no. 12 (December 2000): 1347–52;

H. Yang, "Risk Factors for Gallstone Formation during Rapid Loss of Weight," *Dig Dis Sci* 37, no. 6 (June 1992): 912–18;

C. W. Ko, "Biliary Sludge," *Ann Intern Med* 16, no. 130 (February 1999): 301–11.

Only10 percent develop symptoms within the first five years and 20 percent . . .:

D. E. Howard, "Nonsurgical Management of Gallstone Disease," *Gastroenterol Clin North Am* 28, no. 1 (March 1999): 133–44.

Leave asymptomatic stones alone. Risk of death and disability is greater with immediate surgery:

J. N. Aucott, "Management of Gallstones in Diabetic Patients," *Arch Intern Med* 153, no. 9 (May 1993): 1053–58;

D. F. Ransohoff, "Treatment of Gallstones," *Ann Intern Med* 119 (7 Pt 1) (October 1993): 606–19;

R. Picci et al., "Therapy of Asymptomatic Gallstones: Indications and Limits," *Chir Ital* 57, no. 1 (January–February 2005): 35–45;

A. W. Meshikhes, "Asymptomatic Gallstones in the Laparoscopic Era," *J R Coll Surg Edinb* 47, no. 6 (December 2002): 742–48;

J. Zubler et al., "Natural History of Asymptomatic Gallstones in Family Practice Office Practices, *Arch Fam Med* 7, no. 3 (May–June 1998): 230–33.

Time-honored treatment of gallbladder pain with a low-fat diet:

University of Virginia Health System, "Liver, Biliary & Pancreatic Disorders: Cholecystitis" http://www.healthsystem.virginia.edu/ uvahealth/adult_liver/ chole.cfm and "Gallbladder Disease" http://www.netdoctor.co.uk/diseases/ facts/gallbladderdisease.htm

Risk of gallbladder cancer with asymptomatic gallstones is extremely small;

E. C. Lazcano-Ponce et al., "Epidemiology and Molecular Pathology of Gallbladder Cancer," *CA Cancer J Clin* 51, no. 6 (November–December 2001): 349–64.

Diarrhea after gallbladder surgery;

L. J. O'Donnell, Post-cholecystectomy "Diarrhea: A Running Commentary," *Gut* 45, no. 6 (December 1999): 796–97.

More right-sided colon cancer after gallbladder surgery:

J. Lagergren, "Intestinal Cancer after Cholecystectomy: Is Bile Involved in Carcinogenesis?" *Gastroenterology* 121, no. 3 (September 2001): 542–47.

Treatment of colitis due to bile acids with cholestyramine and colestipol:

K. A. Ung et al., "Role of Bile Acids and Bile Acid Binding Agents in Patients with Collagenous Colitis," *Gut* 46, no. 2 (February 2000): 170–75.

CDCA with UDCA has about a 50 percent success rate in dissolving stones:

M. L. Petroni, "Ursodeoxycholic Acid Alone or with Chenodeoxycholic Acid for Dissolution of Cholesterol Gallstones: A Randomized Multicentre Trial, The British Italian Gallstone Study Group, *Aliment Pharmacol Ther* 15, no. 1 (January 2001): 123–28.

With the addition of cholesterol-lowering medications, Actigall therapy more effective:

S. Tazuma, "A Combination Therapy with Simvastatin and Ursodeoxycholic Acid is More Effective for Cholesterol Gallstone Dissolution than is Ursodeoxycholic Acid Monotherapy," *J Clin Gastroenterol* 26, no. 4 (June 1998): 287–91;

K. D. Saunders, "Lovastatin and Gallstone Dissolution: A Preliminary Study," *Surgery* 113, no. 1 (January 1993): 28–35.

A healthy diet helps dissolve gallstones combined with ursodeoxycholic acid:

S. Moran, "Effects of Fiber Administration in the Prevention of Gallstones in Obese Patients on a Reducing Diet: A Clinical Trial," *Rev
Gastroenterol Mex* 62, no. 4 (October–December 1997): 266–72;

D. P. Maudgal, "A Practical Guide to the Nonsurgical Treatment of Gallstones," *Drugs* 41, no. 2 (February 1991): 185–92.

CHAPTER 7

Obesity encourages the progression of liver disease to cirrhosis:

G. Marchesini et al., "Nonalcoholic Fatty Liver Disease and the
Metabolic Syndrome," *Curr Opin Lipidol* 16, no. 4 (Auguat 2005):
421–27;

G. Gasbarrini et al., "Nonalcoholic Fatty Liver Disease: Defining a Common Problem," *Eur Rev Med Pharmacol Sci* 9, no. 5
(September–October 2005): 253–59.

Carbohydrates are the energy sources most easily utilized by the liver:

Y. A. Ilan, "Balanced 5:1 Carbohydrate:Protein Diet: A New Method for
Supplementing Protein to Patients with Chronic Liver Disease," *J
Gastroenterol Hepatol* 15, no. 12 (December 2000): 1436–41.

*Carbohydrate lowers the risk of cirrhosis, whereas saturated fat increases the
risk associated with alcohol consumption:*

G. Corrao, "Interaction Between Dietary Pattern and Alcohol Intake on
the Risk of Liver Cirrhosis," The Provincial Group for the Study of
Chronic Liver Disease, *Rev Epidemiol Sante Publique* 43, no. 1
(1995): 7–17;

G. Corrao, "Exploring the Role of Diet in Modifying the Effect of
Known Disease Determinants: Application to Risk Factors of Liver
Cirrhosis," *Am J Epidemiol* 142, no. 11 (December 1995): 1136–46.

Vegetable protein is more easily tolerated with impaired liver function:

M. Uribe, "Treatment of Chronic Portal—Systemic Encephalopathy with
Vegetable and Animal Protein Diets: A Controlled Crossover Study,"
Dig Dis Sci 27, no. 12 (December 1982): 1109–16;

G. P. Bianchi et al., "Vegetable versus Animal Protein Diet in Cirrhotic
Patients with Chronic Encephalopathy: A Randomized Cross-over
Comparison," *J Intern Med* 233, no. 5 (May 1993): 385–92.

Nonalcoholic fatty liver disease (NAFLD), with prevalence of 10–51 percent:

G. Gasbarrini et al., "Nonalcoholic Fatty Liver Disease: Defining a Common Problem," *Eur Rev Med Pharmacol Sci* 9, no. 5 (September–
October 2005): 253–59.

High fat and oil consumption are associated with an elevation in liver enzymes:

> R. O. Deems, "Relationship between Liver Biochemical Tests and Dietary Intake in Patients with Liver Disease," *J Clin Gastroenterol* 18, no. 4 (June 1994): 304–08.

A ten- to fifteen-pound weight loss is a very effective means of healing the liver:

> T. Ueno, "Therapeutic Effects of Restricted Diet and Exercise in Obese Patients with Fatty Liver," *J Hepatol* 27, no. 1 (July 1997): 103–07;

> S. Eriksson, "Nonalcoholic Steatohepatitis in Obesity: A Reversible Condition," *Acta Med Scand* 220, no. 1 (1986): 83–88;

> E. J. Drenick, "Effect on Hepatic Morphology of Treatment of Obesity by Fasting, Reducing Diets and Small-Bowel Bypass," *N Engl J Med* 282, no. 15 (April 1970): 829–34;

> P. Vajro, "Persistent Hyperaminotransferasemia Resolving After Weight Reduction in Obese Children," *J Pediatr* 125, no. 2 (August 1994): 239–41.

Lancet, patients were treated with Phyllanthus amarus:

> S. P. Thyagarajan, "Effect of Phyllanthus Amarus on Chronic Carriers of Hepatitis B Virus," *Lancet* 2, no. 8614 (October 1988): 764–66.

More recent reviews of the effectiveness of this herb:

> J. B. Calixto, "A Review of the Plants of the Genus Phyllanthus: Their Chemistry, Pharmacology, and Therapeutic Potential," *Med Res Rev* 18, no. 4 (July 1998): 225–58;

> J. Liu, "Genus Phyllanthus for Chronic Hepatitis B Virus Infection: A Systematic Review," *J Viral Hepat* 8, no. 5, (September 2001): 358–66.

Chinese "Jianpi Wenshen recipe" and the Japanese herbal medicine "Sho-saiko-to" for infectious hepatitis:

> J. P. Liu, "Chinese Medicinal Herbs for Asymptomatic Carriers of Hepatitis B Virus Infection," *Cochrane Database Syst Rev*, 2001, no. 2:CD002231;

> M. Yamashiki, "Effects of the Japanese Herbal Medicine 'Sho-saiko-to' (TJ-9) on In Vitro Interleukin-10 Production by Peripheral Blood Mononuclear Cells of Patients with Chronic Hepatitis C," *Hepatology* 25, no. 6 (June 1997): 1390–97.

Milk thistle protects the liver cells against a variety of toxins:

> P. Ferenci, "Randomized Controlled Trial of Silymarin Treatment in Patients with Cirrhosis of the Liver," *J Hepatol* 9, no. 1 (July 1989): 105–13.

Other herbs have also been used to promote liver health:

S. Luper, "A Review of Plants Used in the Treatment of Liver Disease: Part One," *Altern Med Rev* 3, no. 6 (December 1998): 410–21;

S. Luper, "A Review of Plants Used in the Treatment of Liver Disease: Part Two," *Altern Med Rev* 4, no. 3 (June 1999): 178–88;

R. K. Dhiman and Y. K. Chawla, "Herbal Medicines for Liver Diseases," *Dig Dis Sci* 50, no. 10 (October 2005): 1807–12;

J. R. Jacob et al., "Korean Medicinal Plant Extracts Exhibit Antiviral Potency Against Viral Hepatitis," *J Altern Complement Med* 10, no. 6 (December 2004): 1019–26.

CHAPTER 8

Between 16 and 34 percent of children are reported to be constipated:

V. Loening-Baucke, "Constipation in Children," *N Engl J Med* 339, no. 16 (October 1998): 1155–56.

Sixty-five severely constipated children averaging only one bowel movement every three to fifteen days:

G. Iacono, "Intolerance of Cow's Milk and Chronic Constipation in Children," *N Engl J Med* 339, no. 16 (October 1998): 1100–04.

Cow's milk and constipation:

S. Daher et al., "Cow's Milk Protein Intolerance and Chronic Constipation in Children," *Pediatr Allergy Immunol* 12, no. 6 (December 2001): 339–42;

F. Andiran, S. Dayi, and E. Mete, "Cow's Milk Consumption in Constipation and Anal Fissure in Infants and Young Children," *J Paediatr Child Health* 39, no. 5 (July 2003): 329–31;

G. Iacono et al., "Chronic Constipation as a Symptom of Cow Milk Allergy," *J Pediatr* 126, no. 1 (January 1995): 34–39.

Importance of dietary fiber and constipation prevention:

C. A. Edwards and A. M. Parrett, "Dietary Fibre in Infancy and Childhood," *Proc Nutr Soc* 62, no. 1 (February 2003): 17–23;

A. Wisten and T. Messner, "Fruit and Fibre (Pajala Porridge) in the Prevention of Constipation," *Scand J Caring Sci* 19, no. 1 (March 2005): 71–76.

High-fiber diet cures constipation:

R. Taylor, "Management of Constipation: High Fibre Diets Work," *BMJ* 300, no. 6731 (April 1990): 1063–64;

D. Burkitt, "Effect of Dietary Fibre on Stools and the Transit-Times, and Its Role in the Causation of Disease," *Lancet* 2, no. 7792 (December 1972): 1408–12.

Nearly 70 percent on the Atkins diet report constipation:

> E. C. Westman, "Effect of 6-Month Adherence to a Very Low Carbohy-
> drate Diet Program," *Am J Med* 113, no. 1 (July 2002): 30–36.

Exercise and drinking more water have questionable benefits:

> H. P. Peters, "Potential Benefits and Hazards of Physical Activity and
> Exercise on the Gastrointestinal Tract," *Gut* 48, no. 3 (March 2001):
> 435–39;

> B. D. Chung, "Effect of Increased Fluid Intake on Stool Output in Nor-
> mal Healthy Volunteers," *J Clin Gastroenterol* 28, no. 1 (January
> 1999): 29–32;

> M. Anti, "Water Supplementation Enhances the Effect of High-Fiber
> Diet on Stool Frequency and Laxative Consumption in Adult
> Patients with Functional Constipation," *Hepatogastroenterology* 45,
> no. 21 (May–June 1998): 727–32.

Wheat bran decreases risk of developing colon cancer:

> F. Macrae, "Wheat Bran Fiber and Development of Adenomatous
> Polyps: Evidence from Randomized, Controlled Clinical Trials," *Am
> J Med* 106, no. 1A (January 1999): 38S–42S;

> L. R. Ferguson, "Protection Against Cancer by Wheat Bran: Role of
> Dietary Fibre and Phytochemicals," *Eur J Cancer Prev* 8, no. 1 (Feb-
> ruary 1999): 17–25.

Fruits like prunes and kiwifruit promote bowel movements:

> E. C. Rush, "Kiwifruit Promotes Laxation in the Elderly," *Asia Pac J Clin
> Nutr* 11, no. 2 (2002): 164–68;

> M. Stacewicz-Sapuntzakis, "Chemical Composition and Potential Health
> Effects of Prunes: A Functional Food?" *Crit Rev Food Sci Nutr* 41,
> no. 4 (May 2001): 251–86.

Fiber supplements (PHGG) and wheat bran improve IBS symptoms:

> G. C. Parisi, "High-Fiber Diet Supplementation in Patients with Irritable
> Bowel Syndrome (IBS): A Multicenter Randomized, Open Trial Com-
> parison Between Wheat Bran Diet and Partially Hydrolyzed Guar
> Gum (PHGG)," *Dig Dis Sci* 47, no. 8 (August 2002): 1697–704.

Flaxseeds stimulate bowel function:

> S. C. Cunnane, "Nutritional Attributes of Traditional Flaxseed in
> Healthy Young Adults," *Am J Clin Nutr* 61, no. 1 (January 1995):
> 62–68.

Flaxseeds may also reduce the risk for colon cancer:

> M. Serraino, "Flaxseed Supplementation and Early Markers of Colon
> Carcinogenesis," *Cancer Lett* 63, no. 2 (April 1992): 159–65.

CHAPTER 9

Denis Burkitt, "the fiber man" and McDougall's hero:

A. Ginsberg, "The Fiber Controversy," *Dig Dis*, February 1976, no. 21:103–112;

R. S. Oeppen, "Denis Parsons Burkitt (1911–1993)," *Br J Oral Maxillofac Surg* 41, no. 4 (August 2003): 235;

J. A. Story and D. Kritchevsky, "Denis Parsons Burkitt (1911–1993)," *J Nutr* 124, no. 9 (September 1994): 1551–54.

Modern diseases are rare in underdeveloped populations due to a more healthful diet:

A. Walker, "Epidemiology of Noninfective Intestinal Diseases in Various Ethnic Groups in South Africa," *Isr J Med Sci* 15, no. 4 (April 1979): 309–13;

I. Segal, "Physiological Small Bowel Malabsorption of Carbohydrates Protects Against Large Bowel Diseases in Africans," *J Gastroenterol Hepatol* 17, no. 3 (March 2002): 249–52;

I. Segal, "Persistent Low Prevalence of Western Digestive Diseases in Africa: Confounding Aetiological Factors," *Gut* 48, no. 5 (May 2001): 730–32;

M. Njelekela et al., "Nutritional Variation and Cardiovascular Risk Factors in Tanzania—Rural–Urban Difference," *S Afr Med J* 93, no. 4 (April 2003): 295–99.

Appendicitis is from the Western diet:

G.D. Friedman, "Appendectomy, Appendicitis, and Large Bowel Cancer," *Cancer Res* 50, no. 23 (December 1990): 7549–51;

D. Burkitt, "The Aetiology of Appendicitis," *Br J Surg* 58, no. 9 (September 1971): 695–99;

A. Walker, "Appendicitis, Fibre Intake and Bowel Behaviour in Ethnic Groups in South Africa," *Postgrad Med J* 49, no. 570 (April 1973): 243–49.

The incidence of appendicitis is increasing among Africans as their diet changes:

S. B. Naaeder, "Acute Appendicitis and Dietary Fibre Intake," *West Afr J Med* 17, no. 4 (December 1998): 264–67.

Denis Burkitt never saw diverticular disease among the natives:

J. Simpson, "Pathogenesis of Colonic Diverticula," *Br J Surg* 89, no. 5 (May 2002): 546–54;

N. Painter, "Diverticular Disease of the Colon: A 20th Century Problem," *Clin Gastroenterol* 4, no. 1 (January 1975): 3–21.

The Law of Laplace says contractions at small diameters cause high pressures:

T. Young-Fadok, "Epidemiology and Pathophysiology of Colonic Diverticular Disease," http://www.uptodate.com/patient_info/topicpages/topics/6088F9.asp

Years of elevated pressures produce ruptures in the walls of the intestine, diverticula:

W. H. Aldoori, "A Prospective Study of Dietary Fiber Types and Symptomatic Diverticular Disease in Men," *J Nutr* 128, no. 4 (April 1998): 714–19.

Switching to a high-fiber diet will greatly reduce the risk of future bleeding and infection:

A. L. Leahy, "High Fibre Diet in Symptomatic Diverticular Disease of the Colon," *Ann R Coll Surg Engl* 67, no. 3 (May 1985): 173–74;

M. Eastwood, "Colonic Diverticula," *Proc Nutr Soc* 62, no. 1 (February 2003): 31–36.

Nuts and seeds get caught in diverticula and cause diverticulitis is unsupported:

W. G. Thompson, "Diverticula, Seeds and Nuts," *Digestive Health Matters*, Summer 2003.

Diets low in fiber cause hemorrhoids by creating high pressure in the veins in the anus:

D. Burkitt, "Varicose Veins, Deep Vein Thrombosis, and Haemorrhoids: Epidemiology and Suggested Aetiology," *Br Med J* 2, no. 813 (June 1972): 556–61;

P. Haas, "The Prevalence of Hemorrhoids," *Dis Colon Rectum* 26, no. 7 (July 1983): 435–39;

J. F. Johanson, and A. Sonnenberg, "The Prevalence of Hemorrhoids and Chronic Constipation: An Epidemiologic Study," *Gastroenterology* 98, no. 2 (February 1990): 380–86;

D. Burkitt, "A Deficiency of Dietary Fiber May Be One Cause of Certain Colonic and Venous Disorders," *Am J Dig Dis* 21, no. 2 (February 1976): 104–08.

Africans have switched to a modern diet; now one-fifth have hemorrhoids:

S. W. Ogendo, "A Study of Haemorrhoids As Seen at the Kenyatta National Hospital with Special Reference to Asymptomatic Haemorrhoids," *East Afr Med J* 68, no. 5 (May 1991): 340–47.

Varicose veins are caused by straining:

S. W. Ogendo, "A Study of Haemorrhoids as Seen at the Kenyatta National Hospital with Special Reference to Asymptomatic Haemorrhoids," *East Afr Med J* 68, no. 5 (May 1991): 340–47;

D. Burkitt, "Varicose Veins, Deep Vein Thrombosis, and Haemorrhoids: Epidemiology and Suggested Aetiology," *Br Med J* 2, no. 813 (June 1972): 556–61.

Constipation damages the LES and causes hiatus hernia:

S. J. Sontag, "Defining GERD," *Yale J Biol Med* 72, no. 2–3 (March–June 1999): 69–80;

D. P. Burkitt, "Hiatus Hernia: Is It Preventable?" *Am J Clin Nutr* 34, no. 3 (March 1981): 428–31;

J. P. Capron et al., "Evidence for an Association Between Cholelithiasis and Hiatus Hernia," *Lancet* 2, no. 8085 (August 1978): 329–31.

Prolapsed uterus from constipation:

C. J. Klingele et al., "Pelvic Organ Prolapse in Defecatory Disorders," *Obstet Gynecol* 106, no. 2 (August 2005): 315–20.

CHAPTER 10

Problems with Lotronex and Zelnorm:

R. H. Palmer, "Alosetron for Irritable Bowel Syndrome: Risks of Using Alosetron Are Still Unknown," *BMJ* 326, no. 7379 (January 2003): 51;

J. P. Shapiro, "A Pill Turned Bitter: How a Quest for a Blockbuster Drug Went Fatally Wrong," *US News World Rep,* 129, no. 23 (December 2000): 54–56.

Food intolerances indicated in as much as 58 percent of IBS cases:

S. Zar, "Food Hypersensitivity and Irritable Bowel Syndrome," *Aliment Pharmacol Ther* 15, no. 4 (April 2001): 439–49;

A. N. Niec, "Are Adverse Food Reactions Linked to Irritable Bowel Syndrome?" *Am J Gastroenterol* 93, no. 11 (November 1998): 2184–90;

V. A. Jones, "Food Intolerance: A Major Factor in the Pathogenesis of Irritable Bowel Syndrome," *Lancet* 2, no. 8308 (November 1982): 1115–17;

R. Nanda, "Food Intolerance and the Irritable Bowel Syndrome," *Gut* 30, no. 8 (August 1989): 1099–104.

Improvement of symptoms of IBS simply by adding fiber to the diet:

A. P. Manning, "Wheat Fibre and Irritable Bowel Syndrome: A Controlled Trial," *Lancet* 2, no. 8035 (August 1977): 417–18;

J. P. Lambert, "The Value of Prescribed 'High-fibre' Diets for the Treatment of the Irritable Bowel Syndrome," *Eur J Clin Nutr* 45, no. 12 (December 1991): 601–09;

G. C. Parisi, "High-fiber Diet Supplementation in Patients with Irritable Bowel Syndrome (IBS): A Multicenter, Randomized, Open Trial Comparison Between Wheat Bran Diet and Partially Hydrolyzed Guar Gum (PHGG)," *Dig Dis Sci* 47, no. 8 (August 2002): 1697–704.

IBS treated with probiotics:

K. Niedzielin, "A Controlled, Double-blind, Randomized Study on the Efficacy of *Lactobacillus Plantarum* 299V in Patients with Irritable Bowel Syndrome," *Eur J Gastroenterol Hepatol* 13, no. 10 (October 2001): 1143–47;

G. Bazzocchi, "Intestinal Microflora and Oral Bacteriotherapy in Irritable Bowel Syndrome," *Dig Liver Dis* 34, Suppl 2 (September 2002): S48–53;

P. Gionchetti, "Oral Bacteriotherapy as Maintenance Treatment in Patients with Chronic Pouchitis: A Double-Blind, Placebo-Controlled Trial," *Gastroenterology* 119, no. 2 (August 2000): 305–09.

About 10 percent of people with IBS will also have CD:

G. Robins and P. D. Howdle, "Advances in Celiac Disease," *Curr Opin Gastroenterol* 21, no. 2 (March 2005): 152–61.

Breast-feeding and the introduction of gluten after the first three months reduces future risk:

J. M. Norris et al., "Risk of Celiac Disease Autoimmunity and Timing of Gluten Introduction in the Diet of Infants at Increased Risk of Disease," *JAMA* 293, no. 19 (May 2005): 2343–51.

Health problems common with CD:

A. Alaedini and P. H. Green, "Narrative Review: Celiac Disease: Understanding a Complex Autoimmune Disorder," *Ann Intern Med* 142, no. 4 (February 2005): 289–98;

P. H. Green and B. Jabri, "Coeliac Disease," *Lancet* 362, no. 9381 (August 2003): 383–91.

T. T. Macdonald and G. Monteleone, "Immunity, Inflammation, and Allergy in the Gut," *Science* 307, no. 5717 (March 2005): 1920–25;

M. Viljamaa et al., "Coeliac Disease, Autoimmune Diseases and Gluten Exposure," *Scand J Gastroenterol* 40, no. 4 (April 2005): 437–43;

E. Millward et al., "Gluten- and Casein-free Diets for Autistic Spectrum Disorder," *Cochrane Database Syst Rev*, 2004, no. 2:CD003498;

W. Eaton et al., "Coeliac Disease and Schizophrenia: Population Based Case Control Study with Linkage of Danish National Registers," *BMJ* 328, no. 7437 (February 2004): 438–39.

Offending foods for CD:

> P. J. Ciclitira, H. J. Ellis, and K. E. Lundin, "Gluten-free Diet: What Is Toxic?" *Best Pract Res Clin Gastroenterol* 19, no. 3 (June 2005): 359–71.

Oats may be troublesome:

> H. Arentz-Hansen et al., "The Molecular Basis for Oat Intolerance in Patients with Celiac Disease," *PLoS Med* 1, no. 1 (October 2004): e1.

IBD is found exclusively in societies where people consume a Western diet:

> K. Karlinger, "The Epidemiology and the Pathogenesis of Inflammatory Bowel Disease," *Eur J Radiol* 35, no. 3 (September 2000): 154–67.

Patients with IBD are more likely to consume meat, milk, fat, and refined food, and less likely to consume fruits and vegetables:

> K. D. Cashman and F. Shanahan, "Is Nutrition an Aetiological Factor for Inflammatory Bowel Disease?" *Eur J Gastroenterol Hepatol* 15, no. 6 (June 2003): 607–13;

> A. Tragnone, "Dietary Habits as Risk Factors for Inflammatory Bowel Disease," *Eur J Gastroenterol Hepatol* 7, no. 1 (January 1995): 47–51;

> R. Wright, "Circulating Antibodies to Dietary Proteins in Ulcerative Colitis," *Br Med J*, 1965, 2:142–44;

> N. Mahmud, "The Urban Diet and Crohn's Disease: Is There a Relationship?" *Eur J Gastroenterol Hepatol* 13, no. 2 (February 2001): 93–95;

> J. W. Brandes, "Sugar Free Diet: A New Perspective in the Treatment of Crohn Disease? A Randomized, Control Study," *Gastroenterol* 19, no. 1 (January 1981): 1–12.

Those with UC are likely to have symptoms induced by cow's milk:

> S. M. Samuelsson, "Risk Factors for Extensive Ulcerative Colitis and Ulcerative Proctitis: A Population Based Case-Control Study," *Gut* 32, no. 12 (December 1991): 1526–30.

In Japan, higher fat diets were associated with 2.5 times the risk of IBD:

> N. Sakamoto et al., Epidemiology Group of the Research Committee on Inflammatory Bowel Disease in Japan, "Dietary Risk Factors for Inflammatory Bowel Disease: A Multicenter Case-Control Study in Japan," *Inflamm Bowel Dis* 11, no. 2 (February 2005): 154–63.

Sulfur compounds may also play an important role in the cause of IBD:

> E. Magee E, "A Nutritional Component to Inflammatory Bowel Disease: The Contribution of Meat to Fecal Sulfide Excretion," *Nutrition* 15, no. 3 (March 1999): 244–46;

> J. Levine, "Fecal Hydrogen Sulfide Production in Ulcerative Colitis," *Am J Gastroenterol* 93, no. 1 (January 1998): 83–87;

W. Roediger, "Sulphide Impairment of Substrate Oxidation in Rat Colonocytes: A Biochemical Basis for Ulcerative Colitis?" *Clin Sci (Lond)* 85, no. 5 (November 1993): 623–27.

Elemental diets relieve acute flare-ups of Crohn's disease and are more effective without milk:

M. H. Giaffer, "Controlled Trial of Polymeric versus Elemental Diet in Treatment of Active Crohn's Disease," *Lancet* 335, no. 8603 (April 1990): 816–19.

Dietary fats also reduce the benefits of an elemental diet:

T. Bamba et al., "Dietary Fat Attenuates the Benefits of an Elemental Diet in Active Crohn's Disease: A Randomized, Controlled Trial," *Eur J Gastroenterol Hepatol* 15, no. 2 (February 2003): 151–17.

Two-thirds of patients treated with this diet were well after two years:

V. A. Jones, "Crohn's Disease: Maintenance of Remission by Diet," *Lancet* 2, no. 8448 (July 1985): 177–80.

Eighty-four percent of CD patients achieved remission after two weeks of following an elimination diet:

A. M. Riordan, "Treatment of Active Crohn's Disease by Exclusion Diet: East Anglian Multicentre Controlled Trial," *Lancet* 342, no. 8880 (November 1993): 1131–34.

CD patients find relief from diarrhea overnight on a low-fat diet:

H. Andersson, "Fat-reduced Diet in the Symptomatic Treatment of Patients with Ileopathy," *Nutr Metab* 17, no. 2 (1974): 102–11.

Many early studies have shown patients with UC and CD greatly benefit from a low-fat, plant-based diet:

S. Candy, "The Value of an Elimination Diet in the Management of Patients with Ulcerative Colitis," *S Afr Med J* 85, no. 11 (November 1993): 1176–79.

R. Wright, "A Controlled Therapeutic Trial of Various Diets in Ulcerative Colitis," *Br Med J*, 1965, 22:138–41;

E. M. Workman, "Diet in the Management of Crohn's Disease," *Hum Nutr Appl Nutr* 38, no. 6 (December 1984): 469–73;

K. W. Heaton, "Treatment of Crohn's Disease with an Unrefined-Carbohydrate, Fibre-Rich Diet," *Br Med J* 2, no. 6193 (September 1979): 764–66;

S. Truelove, "Ulcerative Colitis Provoked by Milk," *Br Med J*, 1961, 1:154;

R. Wright, "Controlled Therapeutic Trial of Various Diets in Ulcerative Colitis," *Br Med J*, 1965, 2:138.

CHAPTER 11

Approximately 35 percent of people on the Western diet have colon polyps:

> R. Midgley, "Colorectal Cancer," *Lancet* 353, 9150 (January 1999): 391–409.

Transition time from the earliest changes to cancer takes on average ten to fifteen years:

> S. J. Winawer, "Natural History of Colorectal Cancer," *Am J Med* 106, no. 1A (January 1999): 3S–6S.

Researchers uncovered a fifty-fold variation in the incidence of colon cancer worldwide:

> R. Maric, "Meat Intake, Heterocyclic Amines, and Colon Cancer," *Am J Gastroenterol* 95, no. 12 (December 2000): 3683–84.

Polyps have been shown to regress and disappear when the fecal material is diverted:

> S. M. Feinberg, "Spontaneous Resolution of Rectal Polyps in Patients with Familial Polyposis Following Abdominal Colectomy and Ileo-rectal Anastomosis," *Dis Colon Rectum* 31, no. 3 (March 1988): 169–75.

Burkitt observed that African blacks had virtually no risk of death from colon cancer:

> D. Burkitt, "Epidemiology of Cancer of the Colon and Rectum," *Cancer* 28, no. 1 (July 1971): 3–13;

> S. O'Keefe, "Rarity of Colon Cancer in Africans Is Associated with Low Animal Product Consumption, Not Fiber," *Am J Gastroenterol* 94, no. 5 (May 1999): 1373–80.

Animal fat, cholesterol, meat protein, and lack of plant foods are cancer- and polyp-promoting:

> M. Shike, "Diet and Lifestyle in the Prevention of Colorectal Cancer: An Overview," *Am J Med* 106, no. 1A (January 1999): 11S–15S;

> H. P. Hoensch, and W. Kirch, "Potential Role of Flavonoids in the Prevention of Intestinal Neoplasia: A Review of Their Mode of Action and Their Clinical Perspectives," *Int J Gastrointest Cancer* 35, no. 3 (2005): 187–95.

Even chicken and fish are cancer promoting:

> P. N. Singh, "Dietary Risk Factors for Colon Cancer in a Low-Risk Population," *Am J Epidemiol* 148, no. 8 (October 1998): 761–74.

Hydrogenated fats may be especially cancer-promoting:

> M. L. Slattery, "Trans-fatty Acids and Colon Cancer," *Nutr Cancer* 39, no. 2 (2001): 170–75.

Dietary fiber contributes to a healthy colon and reduces colon cancer risk:

Y. Kim, "AGA Technical Review: Impact of Dietary Fiber on Colon Cancer Occurrence," *Gastroenterology* 118, no. 6 (June 2000): 1235–57;

B. S. Reddy, "Role of Dietary Fiber in Colon Cancer: An Overview," *Am J Med* 106, no. 1A (January 1999): 16S–19S.

Increase fiber intake by 13 grams, decrease colon cancer by 31 percent:

G. R. Howe, "Dietary Intake of Fiber and Decreased Risk of Cancers of the Colon and Rectum: Evidence from the Combined Analysis of 13 Case-Control Studies," *J Natl Cancer Inst* 84, no. 24 (December 1992): 1887–96.

Australian Polyp Prevention Project, with wheat bran reduced polyp recurrence:

R. MacLennan, "Randomized Trial of Intake of Fat, Fiber, and Beta Carotene to Prevent Colorectal Adenomas: The Australian Polyp Prevention Project," *J Natl Cancer Inst* 87, no. 23 (December 1995):1760–66.

The time required for transition from a normal colon to cancer is between twenty-five and thirty-five years:

I. Bhattacharya, "Screening Colonoscopy: The Cost of Common Sense," *Lancet*, 1966, 347:1744;

B. Morson, "Genesis of Colonrectal Cancer," *Clin Gastroenterol*, 1976, 15:505;

S. Stryker, "Natural History of Untreated Colonic Polyps," *Gastroenterology*, 1987, 93:1009.

An effective way to screen would be to do one exam between the ages of fifty-five and sixty:

W. Atkin, "Prevention of Colonrectal Cancer by Once-Only Sigmoidoscopy," *Lancet*, 1993, 341:736;

D. Lieberman, "Cost-Effectiveness Model for Colon Cancer Screening," *Gastroenterology*, 1995, 109:1781;

J. Selby, "Screening Sigmoidoscopy for Colorrectal Cancer: Commentary," *Lancet*, 1993, 341:728.

These tests miss 20 to 50 percent of colon cancers and up to 80 percent of polyps:

M. Pignone, "Screening for Colorectal Cancer in Adults at Average Risk: A Summary of the Evidence for the U.S. Preventive Services Task Force," *Ann Intern Med* 137, no. 2 (July 2002): 132–41.

Tests lead to anxiety, loss of insurability, social stigma, and injury:

K. Marshall, "Population-Based Fecal Occult Blood Screening for Colon Cancer: Will the Benefits Outweigh the Harm?" *CMAJ* 163, no. 5 (September 2000): 545–46.

Sigmoidoscopy every ten years reduced the risk of fatality by 55 percent:

> J. Selby, "A Case-Control Study of Screening Sigmoidoscopy and Mortal-
> ity from Colorectal Cancer," *N Engl J Med*, 1992, 326:653.

Most gastroenterologists are convinced that this is best for the patient:

> S. J. Winawer, "A Comparison of Colonoscopy and Double-Contrast
> Barium Enema for Surveillance after Polypectomy: National Polyp
> Study Work Group," *N Engl J Med* 342, no. 24 (June 2000):
> 1766–72;

> S. J. Winawer, "Randomized Comparison of Surveillance Intervals after
> Colonoscopic Removal of Newly Diagnosed Adenomatous Polyps:
> The National Polyp Study Workgroup," *N Engl J Med* 328, no. 13
> (April 1993): 901–06.

New England Journal of Medicine reported virtual is equal to optical
colonoscopy:

> P. J. Pickhardt, "Computed Tomographic Virtual Colonoscopy to Screen
> for Colorectal Neoplasia in Asymptomatic Adults," *N Engl J Med*
> 349, no. 23 (December 2003): 2191–200.

My preferred alternative to either kind of colonoscopy is a double-contrast
barium enema/sigmoid:

> A. Chapman, "United States has Recommended Screening for Colon
> Cancer: Why Has Barium Enema Been Suggested?" *BMJ*, 1997,
> 314:1624;

> J. Selby, "A Case-Control Study of Screening Sigmoidoscopy and Mortal-
> ity from Colorectal Cancer," *N Engl J Med*, 1992, 326:653;

> G. Dodd, "The Role of the Barium Enema in the Detection of Colonic
> Neoplasms," *Cancer*, 1992, 70:1272;

> S. Halligan and W. Atkin, "Unbiased Studies are Needed Before Virtual
> Colonoscopy Can Be Dismissed," *Lancet* 365, no. 9456 (January
> 2005): 275–76.

Colonoscopies miss finding polyps 24 percent of time:

> D. Rex, "Colonoscopic Miss Rates of Adenomas Determined by Back-to-
> Back Colonoscopies," *Gastroenterology*, 1997, 112:24.

Polyps have been shown to regress and disappear when the fecal material is
diverted:

> S. M. Feinberg, "Spontaneous Resolution of Rectal Polyps in Patients
> with Familial Polyposis Following Abdominal Colectomy and Ileo-
> rectal Anastomosis," *Dis Colon Rectum* 31, no. 3 (March 1988):
> 169–75.

A low-fat, no cholesterol diet can slow the growth of cancer:

> M. L. Littman, "Effect of Cholesterol-Free, Fat-Free Diet and Hypocho-lesteremic Agents on Growth of Transplantable Animal Tumors," *Cancer Chemother Rep* 50, no. 1 (January–February 1966): 25–45;

> H. W. Chen, "The Role of Cholesterol in Malignancy," *Prog Exp Tumor Res*, 1978, 22:275–316;

> J. P. Cruse, "Dietary Cholesterol Deprivation Improves Survival and Reduces Incidence of Metastatic Colon Cancer in Dimethylhy-drazine-Pretreated Rats," *Gut* 23, no. 7 (July 1982): 594–99.

Statins to lower cholesterol may benefit cancer:

> K. K. Chan, "The Statins as Anticancer Agents," *Clin Cancer Res* 9, no. 1 (January 2003): 10–99;

> V. Brower, "Of Cancer and Cholesterol: Studies Elucidate Anticancer Mechanisms of Statins," *J Natl Cancer Inst* 95, no. 12 (June 2003): 844–46;

> M. A. Shibata, "Comparative Effects of Lovastatin on Mammary and Prostate Oncogenesis in Transgenic Mouse Models," *Carcinogenesis* 24, no. 3 (March 2003): 453–59.

Spontaneous regression of colon cancer:

> A. A. Serpick, "Spontaneous Regression of Colon Carcinoma," *Natl Cancer Inst Monogr*, November 1976, 44:21;

> M. Glasser, "Widespread Adenocarcinoma of the Colon with Survival of 28 Years," *JAMA* 241, no. 23 (June 1979): 2542–43.

CHAPTER 12

Microflora has many important functions:

> F. Guarner and J. R. Malagelada, "Gut Flora in Health and Disease," *Lancet* 361, no. 9356 (February 2003): 512–19.

After colectomy, the ilium takes und hecomes colonized with bacteria:

> S. U. Christl and W. Scheppach, "Metabolic Consequences of Total Colectomy," *Scand J Gastroenterol Suppl*, 1997, 222:20–24.

Newborn is inoculated with organisms from the mother's vagina and bowel:

> R. I. Mackie, A. Sghir, and H. R. Gaskins, "Developmental Microbial Ecology of the Neonatal Gastrointestinal Tract," *Am J Clin Nutr* 69, no. 5 (May 1999): 1035S–1045S.

Bifidobacterium *represent 48 percent of the bacteria in breast-fed infants:*

> F. F. Rubaltelli et al., "Intestinal Flora in Breast- and Bottle-fed Infants, *J Perinat Med* 26, no. 3 (1998): 186–91.

Major alterations in the microflora take place within one to two weeks after a change in diet:

> R. Peltonen et al., "An Uncooked Vegan Diet Shifts the Profile of Human Fecal Microflora: Computerized Analysis of Direct Stool Sample Gas-Liquid Chromatography Profiles of Bacterial Cellular Fatty Acids," *Appl Environ Microbiol* 58, no. 11 (November 1992): 3660–66.

Strict vegetarians (vegans) have higher counts of "friendly" bacteria than do meat-eaters:

> B. S. Reddy, J. H. Weisburger, and E. L. Wynder, "Effects of High Risk and Low Risk Diets for Colon Carcinogenesis on Fecal Microflora and Steroids in Man," *J Nutr* 105, no. 7 (July 1975): 878–84;

> P. Toivanen and E. Eerola, "A Vegan Diet Changes the Intestinal Flora," *Rheumatology* (Oxford) 41, no. 8 (August 2002): 950–51.

Conditions helped by specific kinds of probiotics:

> D. C. Montrose and M. H. Floch, "Probiotics Used in Human Studies," *J Clin Gastroenterol* 39, no. 6 (July 2005): 469–84;

> R. N. Fedorak and K. L. Madsen, "Probiotics and Prebiotics in Gastrointestinal Disorders," *Curr Opin Gastroenterol* 20, no. 2 (March 2004): 146–55;

> S. J. Salminen, M. Gueimonde, and E. Isolauri," Probiotics that Modify Disease Risk," *J Nutr* 135, no. 5 (May 2005): 1294–98;

> R. B. Sartor, "Probiotic Therapy of Intestinal Inflammation and Infections," *Curr Opin Gastroenterol* 21, no. 1 (January 2005): 44–50;

> R. Peltonen et al., "Faecal Microbial Flora and Disease Activity in Rheumatoid Arthritis During a Vegan Diet," *Br J Rheumatol* 36, no. 1 (January 1997): 64–68.

Prebiotics may help prevent colon cancer:

> B. S. Reddy, "Prevention of Colon Cancer by Pre- and Probiotics: Evidence from Laboratory Studies," *Br J Nutr* 80, no. 4 (October 1998): S219–23;

> R. K. Buddington et al., "Dietary Supplement of Neosugar Alters the Fecal Flora and Decreases Activities of Some Reductive Enzymes in Human Subjects," *Am J Clin Nutr* 63, no. 5, (May 1996): 709–16.

Lactobacillus bulgaricus *beneficial effects have not been conclusively proven:*

> O. Adolfsson, S. N. Meydani, and R. M. Russell, "Yogurt and Gut Function," *Am J Clin Nutr* 80, no. 2 (August 2004): 245–56.

Lactobacillus acidophilus bacteria has similar drawbacks:

> J. G. Wheeler et al., "Immune and Clinical Impact of *Lactobacillus Acidophilus* on Asthma," *Ann Allergy Asthma Immunol* 79, no. 3 (September 1997): 229–33.

CHAPTER 13

Flatus facts:

> M. Levitt, "The Relation of Passage of Gas and Abdominal Bloating to Colonic Gas Production," *Ann Intern Med* 124, no. 4 (February 1996): 422–24;

> L. Tomlin, "Investigation of Normal Flatus Production in Healthy Volunteers," *Gut* 32, no. 6 (June 1991): 665–69.

Five healthy men showed that over fifteen times more sulfur is produced from a meat diet than a vegetarian diet:

> E. A. Magee, "Contribution of Dietary Protein to Sulfide Production in the Large Intestine: An In Vitro and a Controlled Feeding Study in Humans," *Am J Clin Nutr* 72, no. 6 (December 2000): 1488–94.

White rice is almost completely absorbed, leaving little indigestible carbohydrate:

> M. Levitt, "H2 Excretion After Ingestion of Complex Carbohydrates," *Gastroenterology* 92, no. 2 (February 1987): 383–89.

Flatus from women has higher concentrations of hydrogen sulfide and greater odor:

> F. Suarez, "Identification of Gases Responsible for the Odour of Human Flatus and Evaluation of a Device Purported to Reduce this Odour," *Gut* 43, no. 1 (July 1998): 100–04.

Toxic effects of sulfur on the colon:

> J. Levine, "Fecal Hydrogen Sulfide Production in Ulcerative Colitis," *Am J Gastroenterol* 93, no. 1 (January 1998): 83–87;

> W. Roediger, "Sulphide Impairment of Substrate Oxidation in Rat Colonocytes: A Biochemical Basis for Ulcerative Colitis?" *Clin Sci* (Lond) 85, no. 5 (November 1993): 623–27;

> S. Christl, "Effect of Sodium Sulfide on Cell Proliferation of Colonic Mucosa," *Gastroenterology*, 1994, 106:A664 (abstr);

> S. L. Gorbach and E. Bengt, Gustafsson memorial lecture, "Function of the Normal Human Microflora," *Scand J Infect Dis Suppl*, 1986, 49:17–30.

The indigestible sugars in legumes are heat stable and resistant to cooking:

H. Oboh, "Effect of Soaking, Cooking and Germination on the Oligosaccharide Content of Selected Nigerian Legume Seeds," *Plant Foods Hum Nutr* 55, no. 2 (2000): 97–110.

Sprouting breaks down carbohydrates and reduces bowel gas:

J. W. East, "Changes in Stachyose, Sucrose, and Monosaccharides During Germination of Soybeans," *Crop Sci*, 1972, 12:7–9.

Beano is effective for reducing gas:

T. G. Ganiats, "Does Beano Prevent Gas?: A Double-Blind Crossover Study of Oral Alpha-galactosidase to Treat Dietary Oligosaccharide Intolerance," *J Fam Pract* 39, no. 5 (November 1994): 441–45.

Activated charcoal is effective for reducing gas:

F. Suarez, "Failure of Activated Charcoal to Reduce the Release of Gases Produced by the Colonic Flora," *Am J Gastroenterol* 94, no. 1 (January 1999): 208–12;

T. Potter, "Activated Charcoal: In Vivo and In Vitro Studies of Effect on Gas Formation," *Gastroenterology* 88, no. 3 (March 1985): 620–24.

Probiotics are effective for reducing gas:

S. Nobaek, "Alteration of Intestinal Microflora Is Associated with Reduction in Abdominal Bloating and Pain in Patients with Irritable Bowel Syndrome," *Am J Gastroenterol* 95, no. 5 (May 2000): 1231–38.

CHAPTER 14

The ancestors of modern humans were believed to live almost exclusively on plant foods:

B. Wood, "Human Evolution: We Are What We Ate," *Nature*, 1999, 400:219–20;

K. Milton, "Back to Basics: Why Foods of Wild Primates Have Relevance for Modern Human Health," *Nutrition* 16, no. 7–8 (July 2000): 480–83;

K. Milton, "Hunter-Gatherer Diets: A Different Perspective," *Am J Clin Nutr* 71, no. 3 (March 2000): 665–67;

M. Nestle, "Animal v. Plant Foods in Human Diets and Health: Is the Historical Record Unequivocal?" *Proc Nutr Soc* 58, no. 2 (May 1999): 211–18;

E. Pennisi, "Did Cooked Tubers Spur the Evolution of Big Brains?" *Science* 283, no. 5410 (March 1999): 2004–05.

Biologists at Wayne State University School of Medicine say we are like chimps:

> "Chimpanzees are also in the Homo species" http://news.national
> geographic.com/news/2003/05/0520_030520_chimpanzees.html

Nature reported: Of the 3 billion genes of human and chimpanzees, 96 percent are identical:

> D. Carina, "Chimp Genome: Branching Out," *Nature*, September 2005,
> no. 437:17–19.

Anatomic and physiologic comparisons of humans that make us herbivores:

> K. Milton, "Back to Basics: Why Foods of Wild Primates Have Rele-
> vance for Modern Human Health," *Nutrition* 16, no. 7–8
> (July–August 2000): 480–83;
>
> K. Milton, "Hunter-Gatherer Diets: A Different Perspective," *Am J Clin
> Nutr* 71, no. 3 (March 2000): 665–67;
>
> K. Milton, "A Hypothesis to Explain the Role of Meat-Eating in Human
> Evolution," *Evol Anthropol*, 1999, 8:11–21;
>
> K. J. Carpenter, "Protein Requirements of Adults from an Evolutionary
> Perspective," *Am J Clin Nutr* 55, no. 5 (May 1992): 913–17;
>
> W. Collens, "Phylogenetic Aspects of the Cause of Human Atheroscle-
> rotic Disease," *Circulation* Suppl II, 31–32 (1965): II–7;
>
> C. Prosser, *Comparative Animal Physiology*, 2nd ed. (Philadelphia: W. B.
> Saunders, 1961), 116;
>
> E. Nasset, "Movements of the Small Intestine," P Bard, *Medical Physiolo-
> gy*, 11th ed. (St. Louis: C. V. Mosby, 1961), 440;
>
> *What's Wrong with Eating Meat?* (New Delhi: Ananda Marga Publica-
> tions, 1977).

Four thousand people die each year in the United States from "café coronary":

> H. Heimlich, "A Life-Saving Maneuver to Prevent Food-Choking,"
> *JAMA*, 1975, 234:398–401.

The tongue of a carnivore does not have sensors for carbohydrates but for ani-mal proteins:

> X. Li et al., "Pseudogenization of a Sweet-Receptor Gene Accounts
> for Cats' Indifference toward Sugar," *PLoS Genet* 1, no. 1 (July
> 2005): e3.

Cholesterol overwhelms a plant-eater's liver:

> J. Dietschy, "Regulation of Cholesterol Metabolism," *N Engl J Med* 282,
> no. 22 (May 1970): 1241–49.

Our requirements are for plant nutrients:

K. Milton, "Hunter-Gatherer Diets: A Different Perspective," *Am J Clin Nutr* 71, no. 3 (March 2000): 665–67;

K. Milton, "A Hypothesis to Explain the Role of Meat-Eating in Human Evolution," *Evol Anthropol*, 1999, no. 8:11–21;

K. J. Carpenter, "Protein Requirements of Adults from an Evolutionary Perspective," *Am J Clin Nutr* 55, no. 5 (May 1992): 913–17.

Human males have seminal vesicles—no other meat-eating animal has these important semen collecting-pouches:

D. Coffey, "Similarities of Prostate and Breast Cancer: Evolution, Diet, and Estrogens," *Urology*, Suppl 1, 4, no. 57 (2001): 31–38.

Vegetarian diet ideal for human health:

M. Segasothy, "Vegetarian Diet: Panacea for Modern Lifestyle?" *Q J Med*, 1999, no. 92:531–44.

References

Acalovschi, M. 2001. Cholesterol gallstones: From epidemiology to prevention. *Postgrad Med J* 77 (October) 906:221–29.

Adolfsson, O., Meydani S. N., and Russell R. M. 2004. Yogurt and gut function. *Am J Clin Nutr* 80 (August) 2:245–56.

Alaedini, A., and Green P. H. 2005. Narrative review—Celiac disease: Understanding a complex autoimmune disorder. *Ann Intern Med* 142 (February) (4):289–98.

Alberti, K. G., P. Zimmet, and J. Shaw. IDF Epidemiology Task Force Consensus Group. 2005. The metabolic syndrome: A new worldwide definition. *Lancet* 24–30, 366(9491): 1059–62.

Aldoori, W. H. 1998. A prospective study of dietary fiber types and symptomatic diverticular disease in men. *J Nutr* 128 (April) (4):714–19.

Allen, M. L. 1990. The effect of raw onions on acid reflux and reflux symptoms. *Am J Gastroenterol* 85 (4):377–80.

Andersson, H. 1974. Fat-reduced diet in the symptomatic treatment of patients with ileopathy. *Nutr Metab* 17 (2): 102–11.

Andiran, F., S. Dayi, and E. Mete. 2003. Cow's milk consumption in constipation and anal fissure in infants and young children. *J Paediatr Child Health* 39 (July) 5:329–31.

Anti, M. 1998. Water supplementation enhances the effect of high-fiber diet on stool frequency and laxative consumption in adult patients with functional constipation. *Hepatogastroenterology* 45 (May–June) 21:727–32.

Arentz-Hansen, H., B. Fleckenstein O. Molberg, H. Scott, F. Koning, G. Jung, P. Roepstorff, K. E. Lundin, and L. M. Sollid. 2004. The molecular basis for oat intolerance in patients with celiac disease. *PLoS Med* 1 (October) 1:e1.

Astrup, A., B. Buemann, A. Flint, and A. Raben. 2002. Low-fat diets and energy balance: How does the evidence stand in 2002? *Proc Nutr Soc* 61 (2): 299–309.

Atkin, W. 1993. Prevention of colonrectal cancer by once-only sigmoidoscopy. *Lancet* 341:736.

Aucott, J. N. 1993. Management of gallstones in diabetic patients. *Arch Intern Med* 153 (May) 9:1053–58.

Awano, S., S. Koshimune, E. Kurihara, K. Gohara, A. Sakai, I. Soh, T. Hamasaki, T. Ansai, and T. Takehara. 2004. The assessment of methyl mercaptan: An important clinical marker for the diagnosis of oral malodor. *J Dent* 32 (7): 555–59.

Babidge, W., S. Millard, and W. Roediger. 1998. Sulfides impair short chain fatty acid beta-oxidation at acyl-CoA dehydrogenase level in colonocytes: Implications for ulcerative colitis. *Mol Cell Biochem* 181 (1–2): 117–24.

Babka, J. 1973. On the genesis of heartburn: The effects of specific foods on the lower esophageal sphincter. *Am J Dig Dis* 18 (5): 391–97.

Bamba, T., T. Shimoyama, M. Sasaki, T. Tsujikawa, Y. Fukuda, K. Koganei, et al. 2003. Dietary fat attenuates the benefits of an elemental diet in active Crohn's disease: A randomized, controlled trial. *Eur J Gastroenterol Hepatol* 15 (February) 2:151–57.

Bazzocchi, G. 2002. Intestinal microflora and oral bacteriotherapy in irritable bowel syndrome. *Dig Liver Dis* Suppl. no. 2 (September) 34:S48-53.

Becker, D. 1989. A comparison of high and low fat meals on postprandial esophageal acid exposure. *Am J Gastroenterol* 84 (7): 782–86.

Bhattacharya, I. 1996. Screening colonoscopy: The cost of common sense. *Lancet* 347:1744.

Bianchi, G. P., G. Marchesini, A. Fabbri, A. Rondelli, E. Bugianesi, M. Zoli, and E. Pisi. 1993. Vegetable versus animal protein diet in cirrhotic patients with chronic encephalopathy: A randomized cross-over comparison. *J Intern Med* 233 (May) 5:385–92.

Bolin, T. D. 2000. Heartburn: Community perceptions. *J Gastroenterol Hepatol* 15 (1): 35–39.

Brandes, J. W. 1981. Sugar-free diet: A new perspective in the treatment of Crohn disease?: randomized, control study. *Gastroenterol* 19 (January) 1:1–12.

Briggs, R. 1960. Myocardial infarction in patients treated with Sippy and other high-milk diets: An autopsy study of fifteen hospitals in the USA and Great Britain. *Circulation* 21:538.

Brooks, F. P. 1985. Effect of diet on gastric secretion. *Am J Clin Nutr* Suppl no. 5, 42 (5): 1006–19.

Brower, V. 2003. Of cancer and cholesterol: studies elucidate anticancer mechanisms of statins. *J Natl Cancer Inst* 95 (June) 12:844–6.

Brown, L. M. 2000. Helicobacter pylori: epidemiology and routes of transmission. *Epidemiol Rev* 22 (2): 283–97.

Buddington, R. K., C. H. Williams, S. C. Chen, and S. A. Witherly. 1996. Dietary supplement of neosugar alters the fecal flora and decreases activities of some reductive enzymes in human subjects. *Am J Clin Nutr* 63 (May) 5:709–16.

Burkitt, D. 1971a. The aetiology of appendicitis. *Br J Surg* 58 (September) 9:695–99.

———. 1971b Epidemiology of cancer of the colon and rectum. *Cancer* 28 (July) 1:3–13.

——— 1972a. Effect of dietary fibre on stools and the transit-times, and its role in the causation of disease. *Lancet* 2 (December) 7792:1408—12.

———. 1972b. Varicose veins, deep vein thrombosis, and haemorrhoids: Epidemiology and suggested aetiology. *Br Med J* 2 (June) 813:556–61.

————. 1976. A deficiency of dietary fiber may be one cause of certain colonic and venous disorders. *Am J Dig Dis* 21 (February) 2:104–08.

————. 1981. Hiatus hernia: Is it preventable? *Am J Clin Nutr* 34 (March) 3:428–31.

Bytzer P., and C. O'Morain. 2005. Treatment of *Helicobacter pylori*. *Helicobacter* Suppl. no. 1, 10:40–46.

Calixto, J. B. 1998. A review of the plants of the genus *Phyllanthus*: Their chemistry, pharmacology, and therapeutic potential. *Med Res Rev* 18 (July) 4:225–58.

Candy, S. 1995. The value of an elimination diet in the management of patients with ulcerative colitis. *S Afr Med J* 85 (November) 11:1176–79.

Capron, J. P., H. Payenneville, M. Dumont, J. L. Dupas, and A. Lorriaux. 1978. Evidence for an association between cholelithiasis and hiatus hernia. *Lancet* 2 (August) 8085:329–31.

Carina, D. 2005. Chimp genome: Branching out. *Nature* 437 (September): 17–19.

Carpenter, K. J. 1992. Protein requirements of adults from an evolutionary perspective. *Am J Clin Nutr* 55 (May) 5:913–17.

Cashman, K. D., and F. Shanahan. 2003. Is nutrition an aetiological factor for inflammatory bowel disease? *Eur J Gastroenterol Hepatol* 15 (June) 6:607–13.

Chan, K. K. 2003. The statins as anticancer agents. *Clin Cancer Res* 9 (January) 1:10–19.

Chapman, A. 1997. United States has recommended screening for colon cancer: Why has barium enema been suggested? *BMJ* 314:1624.

Chen, H. W. 1978. The role of cholesterol in malignancy. *Prog Exp Tumor Res* 22:275–316.

Childs, P. 1972. Dietary fat, dyspepsia, diarrhoea, and diabetes. *Br J Surg* 59:669–95.

Christl, S. 1994. Effect of sodium sulfide on cell proliferation of colonic mucosa. *Gastroenterology* 106:A664 (abstr).

Christl, S. U., and W. Scheppach. 1997. Metabolic consequences of total colectomy. *Scand J Gastroenterol* Suppl. 222:20–24.

Chung, B. D. 1999. Effect of increased fluid intake on stool output in normal healthy volunteers. *J Clin Gastroenterol* 28 (January) 1:29–32.

Ciclitira, P. J., H. J. Ellis, and K. E. Lundin. 2005. Gluten-free diet: What is toxic? *Best Pract Res Clin Gastroenterol* 19 (June) 3:359–71.

Clearfield, H. 1991. *Helicobacter pylori*: Aggressor or innocent bystander? *Med Clin North Am* 75 (July) 4:815–29

Coffey, D. 2001. Similarities of prostate and breast cancer: Evolution, diet, and estrogens. *Urology* Suppl. no 1, 4(57): 31–8.

Cohen, S. 1975. Gastric acid secretion and lower-esophageal-sphincter pressure in response to coffee and caffeine. *N Engl J Med* 293 (18): 897–99.

Collens, W. 1965. Phylogenetic Aspects of the Cause of Human Atherosclerotic Disease. *Circulation* Suppl. no. 2, 31–32: II–7.

Corrao, G. 1995. Exploring the role of diet in modifying the effect of known disease determinants: Application to risk factors of liver cirrhosis. *Am J Epidemiol* 142 (December) 11:1136–46.

———. 1995. Interaction between dietary pattern and alcohol intake on the risk of liver cirrhosis. The Provincial Group for the Study of Chronic Liver Disease. *Rev Epidemiol Sante Publique* 43 (1): 7–17.

Cranley, J. P. 1986. Abnormal lower esophageal sphincter pressure responses in patients with orange juice-induced heartburn. *Am J Gastroenterol* 81 (2): 104–06.

Crohn, B. 1920. *Am J Med Sci* 59:70.

Cruse, J. P. 1982. Dietary cholesterol deprivation improves survival and reduces incidence of metastatic colon cancer in dimethylhydrazine-pretreated rats. *Gut* 23 (July) 7:594–99.

Cuevas, A., J. F. Miquel, M. S. Reyes, S. Zanlungo, and F. Nervi. 2004. Diet as a risk factor for cholesterol gallstone disease. *J Am Coll Nutr* 23 (June) 3:187–96.

Cummings, J. H. 1983. Fermentation in the human large intestine: Evidence and implications for health. *Lancet* 1 (8335): 1206–09.

Cunnane, S. C. 1995. Nutritional attributes of traditional flaxseed in healthy young adults. *Am J Clin Nutr* 61 (January) 1:62–68.

Daher S., S. Tahan, D. Sole, C. K. Naspitz, F. R. Da Silva Patricio, U. F. Neto, and M. B. De Morais. 2001. Cow's milk protein intolerance and chronic constipation in children. *Pediatr Allergy Immunol* 12 (December) 6:339–42.

Dalton, P. 2000. Psychophysical and behavioral characteristics of olfactory adaptation. *Chem Senses* 25 (4): 487–92.

Deems, R. O. 1994. Relationship between liver biochemical tests and dietary intake in patients with liver disease. *J Clin Gastroenterol* 18 (June) 4:304–08.

Dhiman, R. K., and Y. K. Chawla. 2005. Herbal medicines for liver diseases. *Dig Dis Sci* 50 (October) 10:1807–12.

Dietschy, J. 1970. Regulation of cholesterol metabolism. *N Engl J Med* 282 (May) 22:1241–49.

Dodd, G. 1992. The role of the barium enema in the detection of colonic neoplasms. *Cancer* 70:1272.

Doll, R., and F. 1954. Pygott. Clinical trial of Robaden and of cabbage juice in the treatment of gastric ulcer. *Lancet* 267 (December) 6850:1200–04.

Dowling, R. 2000. Review: Pathogenesis of gallstones. *Aliment Pharmacol Ther* Suppl. 14 (May) 2:39–47.

Drenick, E. J. 1970. Effect on hepatic morphology of treatment of obesity by fasting, reducing diets and small-bowel bypass. *N Engl J Med* 282 (April) 15:829–34.

Dunn, B. 1997. *Helicobacter pylori. Clin Microbiol Rev* 10 (October) 4:720–41.

East, J. W. 1972. Changes in stachyose, sucrose, and monosaccharides during germination of soybeans. *Crop Sci* 12:7–9.

Eastwood, M. 2003. Colonic diverticula. *Proc Nutr Soc* 62 (February) 1:31–36.

Eaton, W., P. B. Mortensen, E. Agerbo, M. Byrne, O. Mors, and H. Ewald. 2004. Coeliac disease and schizophrenia: population based case control study with linkage of Danish national registers. *BMJ* 328 (February) 7437:438–39.

Edwards, C. A., and A. M. Parrett. 2003. Dietary fibre in infancy and childhood. *Proc Nutr Soc* 62)February) 1:17–23.

Elmstahl, S. 1998. Fermented milk products are associated to ulcer diseases: Results from a cross-sectional population study. *Eur J Clin Nutr* (52):668–74.

Elta, G. H. 1990. Comparison of coffee intake and coffee-induced symptoms in patients with duodenal ulcer, nonulcer dyspepsia, and normal controls. *Am J Gastroenterol* 85 (10): 1339–42.

Eriksson, S. 1986. Nonalcoholic steatohepatitis in obesity: A reversible condition. *Acta Med Scand* 220 (1): 83–88.

Erlinger, S. 2000. Gallstones in obesity and weight loss. *Eur J Gastroenterol Hepatol* 12 (December) 12:1347–52.

Everhart, J. E., F. Yeh, E. T. Lee, M. C. Hill, R. Fabsitz, B. V. Howard, and T. K. Welty. 2002. Prevalence of gallbladder disease in American Indian populations: Findings from the Strong Heart Study. *Hepatology* 35 (June) 6:1507–12.

Everhart, J. E. 1999. Prevalence and ethnic differences in gallbladder disease in the United States. *Gastroenterology* 117 (September) 3:632–39.

Fabry, W., P. Okemo, and R. Ansborg. 1996. Activity of East African medicinal plants against *Helicobacter pylori*. *Chemotherapy* 42:315–317.

Farrow, D. C. 2000. Gastroesophageal reflux disease, use of H2 receptor antagonists, and risk of esophageal and gastric cancer. *Cancer Causes Control* 11 (3): 231–38.

Fedorak, R. N., and K. L. Madsen. 2004. Probiotics and prebiotics in gastrointestinal disorders. *Curr Opin Gastroenterol* 20 (March) 2:146–55.

Feinberg, S. M. 1988. Spontaneous resolution of rectal polyps in patients with familial polyposis following abdominal colectomy and ileorectal anastomosis. *Dis Colon Rectum* 31 (March) 3:169–75.

Ferenci, P. 1989. Randomized controlled trial of silymarin treatment in patients with cirrhosis of the liver. *J Hepatol* 9 (July) 1:105–13.

Ferguson, L. R. 1999. Protection against cancer by wheat bran: role of dietary fibre and phytochemicals. *Eur J Cancer Prev* 8 (February) 1:17–25.

Friedman, G. D. 1990. Appendectomy, appendicitis, and large bowel cancer. *Cancer Res* 50 (December) 23:7549–51.

———. 1993. Natural history of asymptomatic and symptomatic gallstones. *Am J Surg* 165 (April) 4:399–404.

Galan, M. V., A. A. Kishan, and A. I. Silverman. 2004. Oral broccoli sprouts for the treatment of Helicobacter pylori infection. A preliminary report. *Dig Dis Sci* 49 (August) 7–8:1088–90.

Ganiats, T. G. 1994. Does Beano prevent gas? A double-blind crossover study of oral alpha-galactosidase to treat dietary oligosaccharide intolerance. *J Fam Pract* 39 (November) 5:441–5.

Gasbarrini, G., V. Vero, L. Miele, A. Forgione, A. P. Hernandez, A. V. Greco, A. Gasbarrini, and A. Grieco. 2005. Nonalcoholic fatty liver disease: Defining a common problem. *Eur Rev Med Pharmacol Sci* 9 (September– October) 5:253–59.

Giaffer, M. H. 1990. Controlled trial of polymeric versus elemental diet in treatment of active Crohn's disease. *Lancet* 335 (April) 8693:816–19.

Ginsberg, A. 1976. The fiber controversy. *Dig Dis* (February) 21:103–112.

Gionchetti, P. 2000. Oral bacteriotherapy as maintenance treatment in patients with chronic pouchitis: A double-blind, placebo-controlled trial. *Gastroenterology* 119 (August) 2:305–09.

Glasser M. 1979. Widespread adenocarcinoma of the colon with survival of 28 years. *JAMA* 241 (June) 23:2542–43

Glise, H. 1995. Quality of life assessments in the evaluation of gastroesophageal reflux and peptic ulcer disease before, during and after treatment. *Scand J Gastroenterol* Suppl 208:133–35.

Goel, M. S., E. P. McCarthy, R. S. Phillips, and C. C. Wee. 2004. Obesity among US immigrant subgroups by duration of residence. *JAMA* 15;292(23): 2860–67.

Gopal, B., P. Singhal, and S. N. Gaur. 2005. Gastroesophageal reflux disease in bronchial asthma and the response to omeprazole. *Asian Pac J Allergy Immunol* 23(1): 29–34.

Gorbach, S. L., and E. Bengt. 1986. Gustafsson memorial lecture. Function of the normal human microflora. *Scand J Infect Dis* Suppl. 49:17–30.

Graham, D. 1988. Spicy food and the stomach: Evaluation by videoendoscopy. *JAMA* 260:3473–75.

Green, P. H, and B. Jabri. 2003. Coeliac disease. *Lancet* 362 (August) 9381:383–91.

Groen, J. N., and A. J. Smout. 2003. Supra-oesophageal manifestations of gastro-oesophageal reflux disease. *Eur J Gastroenterol Hepatol* 15 (12): 1339–50.

Guarner, F., and J. R. Malagelada. 2003. Gut flora in health and disease. *Lancet* 361 (February) 9356:512–19.

Haas, P. 1983. The prevalence of hemorrhoids. *Dis Colon Rectum* 26 (July) 7:435–39.

Halligan, S., and W. Atkin. 2005. Unbiased studies are needed before virtual colonoscopy can be dismissed. *Lancet* 365 (January) 9456:275–76.

Havlicek, J., S. C. Roberts, and J. Flegr. 2005. *Biol. Lett* doi:10. 1098/rsbl:0332.

Hayes, K. C, A. Livingston, and E. A. Trautwein. 1992. Dietary impact on biliary lipids and gallstones. *Annu Rev Nutr* 12:299–326.

Heaton, K. W. 1979. Treatment of Crohn's disease with an unrefined-carbohydrate, fibre-rich diet. *Br Med J* 2 (September) 6193:764–66.

Heimburger, D. C., V. A. Stallings, and L. Routzahn. 1998. Survey of clinical nutrition training programs for physicians. *Am J Clin Nutr* 68(6): 1174–79.

Heimlich, H. 1975. A Life-Saving Maneuver to Prevent Food-Choking. *JAMA* 234:398–401.

Hoensch, H. P, and W. Kirch. 2005. Potential role of flavonoids in the prevention of intestinal neoplasia: a review of their mode of action and their clinical perspectives. *Int J Gastrointest Cancer* 35(3): 187–95.

Hogan, W. 1972. Ethanol-induced acute esophageal motor dysfunction. *J Appl Physiol* 32(6): 755–60.

———. 2001. Medical treatment of supraesophageal complications of gastroesophageal reflux disease. *Am J Med* 111 Suppl. no. 8A:197S–201S.

Holloway, R. H. 1985. Gastric distention: a mechanism for postprandial gastroesophageal reflux. *Gastroenterology* 89(4): 779–84.

————. 1997. Effect of intraduodenal fat on lower oesophageal sphincter function and gastro-oesophageal reflux. *Gut* 40(4): 449–53.

Holzer, P. 1988. Stimulation of afferant nerve endings by intragastric capsaicin protects against ethanol-induced damage of gastric mucosa. *Neuroscience* 27:981–87.

————. 1989. Intragastric capsaicin protects against aspirin-induced lesion formation and bleeding in rat gastric mucosa. *Gastroenterlogy* 96(6): 1425–33.

Howard, D. E. 1999. Nonsurgical management of gallstone disease. *Gastroenterol Clin North Am* 28 (March) 1:133–44.

Howe, G. R. 1992. Dietary intake of fiber and decreased risk of cancers of the colon and rectum: Evidence from the combined analysis of 13 case-control studies. *J Natl Cancer Inst* 84 (December) 24:1887–96.

Iacono, G, A. Carroccio, F. Cavataio, G. Montalto, M. D. Cantarero, and A. Notarbartolo. 1995. Chronic constipation as a symptom of cow milk allergy. *J Pediatr* 126 (January) 1:34–39.

Iacono, G. 1998. Intolerance of cow's milk and chronic constipation in children. *N Engl J Med* 339 (October) 16:1100–04.

Ilan, Y. 2000. A balanced 5:1 carbohydrate:protein diet: a new method for supplementing protein to patients with chronic liver disease. *J Gastroenterol Hepatol* 15 (December) 12:1436–41.

Ippoliti, A. F. 1976. The effect of various forms of milk on gastric-acid secretion: Studies in patients with duodenal ulcer and normal subjects. *Ann Intern Med* 84(3): 286–89.

Jacob, J. R., B. E. Korba, J. E. You, B. C. Tennant, and Y. H. Kim. 2004. Korean medicinal plant extracts exhibit antiviral potency against viral hepatitis. *J Altern Complement Med* 10 (December) 6:1019–26.

James, P. T. 2004. Obesity: the worldwide epidemic. *Clin Dermatol* 22(4): 276–80.

Johanson, J. F, and A. Sonnenberg. 1990. The prevalence of hemorrhoids and chronic constipation: An epidemiologic study. *Gastroenterology* 98 (February) 2:380–86.

Jones, V. A. 1982. Food intolerance: A major factor in the pathogenesis of irritable bowel syndrome. *Lancet* 2 (November) 8308:1115–17.

————. 1985. Crohn's disease: Maintenance of remission by diet. *Lancet* 2 (July) 8448:177–80.

Kaplan, M. C., N. Huguet, J. T. Newsom, and B. H. McFarland. 2004. The association between length of residence and obesity among Hispanic immigrants. *Am J Prev Med* 27(4): 323–26.

Karlinger K. 2000. The epidemiology and the pathogenesis of inflammatory bowel disease. *Eur J Radiol* 35 (September) 3:154–67.

Katz, J. 2001. Inflammation, periodontitis, and coronary heart disease. *Lancet* 358:303.

Kim, Y. 2000. AGA technical review: Impact of dietary fiber on colon cancer occurrence. *Gastroenterology* 118 (June) 6:1235–57.

Klingele, C. J., A. E. Bharucha, J. G. Fletcher, J. B. Gebhart, S. G. Riederer, and A. R. Zinsmeister. 2005. Pelvic organ prolapse in defecatory disorders. *Obstet Gynecol* 106 (August) 2:315–20.

Ko, C. W. 1999. Biliary sludge. *Ann Intern Med* 130 (February) 4(Pt 1): 301–11.

Kratzer, W., R. A. Mason, and V. Kachele. 1999. Prevalence of gallstones in sonographic surveys worldwide. *J Clin Ultrasound* 27 (January) 1:1–7.

Kratzer, W. 1997. Gallstone prevalence in relation to smoking, alcohol, coffee consumption, and nutrition: The Ulm Gallstone Study. *Scand J Gastroenterol* 32 (September) 9:953–58.

Kumar, N. 1984. Do chilies influence healing of duodenal ulcer? *BMJ* 288:1803–04.

Kushner R. F., F. K. Thorp, J. Edwards, R. L. Weinsier, and C. M. Brooks. 1990. Implementing nutrition into the medical curriculum: A user's guide. *Am J Clin Nutr* 52(2): 401–03.

Lagergren, J. 2001. Intestinal cancer after cholecystectomy: Is bile involved in carcinogenesis? *Gastroenterology* 121 (September) 3:542–47.

Lambert, J. P. 1991. The value of prescribed 'high-fibre' diets for the treatment of the irritable bowel syndrome. *Eur J Clin Nutr* 45 (December) 12:601–09.

Larkai, E. N. 1987. Gastroduodenal mucosa and dyspeptic symptoms in arthritic patients during chronic nonsteroidal anti-inflammatory drug use. *Am J Gastroenterol* 82 (November) 11:1153–58.

Lazcano-Ponce, E. C., J. F. Miquel, N. Munoz, R. Herrero, C. Ferrecio, I. I. Wistuba, P. Alonso de Ruiz, G. Aristi Urista, and F. Nervi. 2001. Epidemiology and molecular pathology of gallbladder cancer. *CA Cancer J Clin* 51 (November-December) 6:349–64.

Leahy, A. L. 1985. High fibre diet in symptomatic diverticular disease of the colon. *Ann R Coll Surg Engl* 67 (May) 3:173–74.

Levine, J. 1998. Fecal hydrogen sulfide production in ulcerative colitis. *Am J Gastroenterol* 93 (January) 1:83–87.

Levitt, M. 1987. H2 excretion after ingestion of complex carbohydrates. *Gastroenterology* 92 (February) 2:383–89.

Levitt, M. 1966. The relation of passage of gas an abdominal bloating to colonic gas production. *Ann Intern Med* 124 (February) 4:422–24.

Li, X., W. Li, H. Wang, J. Cao, K. Maehashi, L. Huang, A. A. Bachmanov, D. R. Reed, V. Legrand-Defretin, G. K. Beauchamp, and J. G. Brand. 2005. Pseudogenization of a sweet-receptor gene accounts for cats' indifference toward sugar. *PLoS Genet* 1 (July) 1:e3.

Lieberman, D. 1995. Cost-effectiveness model for colon cancer screening. *Gastroenterology* 109:1781.

Littman, M. L. 1966. Effect of cholesterol-free, fat-free diet and hypocholesteremic agents on growth of transplantable animal tumors. *Cancer Chemother Rep* 50 (January-February) 1:25–45.

Liu, J. 2001. Genus Phyllanthus for chronic hepatitis B virus infection: A systematic review. *J Viral Hepat* 8 (September) 5:358–66.

Liu, J. P. 2001. Chinese medicinal herbs for asymptomatic carriers of hepatitis B virus infection. *Cochrane Database Syst Rev* (2): CD002231.

Loening-Baucke, V. 1998. Constipation in children. *N Engl J Med* 339 (October) 16:1155–56.

Luper, S. 1998. A review of plants used in the treatment of liver disease: Part one. *Altern Med Rev* 3 (December) 6:410–21.

————. 1998. A review of plants used in the treatment of liver disease: Part two. *Altern Med Rev* 4 (June) 3:178–88.

Macdonald, T. T, and G. Monteleone. 2005. Immunity, inflammation, and allergy in the gut. *Science* 307 (March) 5717:1920–25.

Mackie, R. I., A. Sghir, and H. R. Gaskins. 1999. Developmental microbial ecology of the neonatal gastrointestinal tract. *Am J Clin Nutr* 69 (May) 5:1035S–1045S.

MacLennan, R. 1995. Randomized trial of intake of fat, fiber, and beta carotene to prevent colorectal adenomas: The Australian Polyp Prevention Project. *J Natl Cancer Inst* 87 (December) 23:1760–66.

Macrae, F. 1999. Wheat bran fiber and development of adenomatous polyps: Evidence from randomized, controlled clinical trials. *Am J Med* 106 (January) 1A:38S–42S.

Magee, E. 1999. A nutritional component to inflammatory bowel disease: The contribution of meat to fecal sulfide excretion. *Nutrition* 15 (March) 3:244–46.

Magee, E. A. 2000. Contribution of dietary protein to sulfide production in the large intestine: An in vitro and a controlled feeding study in humans. *Am J Clin Nutr* 72 (December) 6:1488–94.

Mahady, G.B. Allixin, a phytoalexin from garlic, inhibits the growth of Helicobacter pylori in vitro. *Am J Gastroenterol* 96 (December) 12:3454–55.

Mahmud, N. 2001. The urban diet and Crohn's disease: Is there a relationship? *Eur J Gastroenterol Hepatol* 13 (February) 2:93–95.

Manning, A. P. 1977. Wheat fibre and irritable bowel syndrome: A controlled trial. *Lancet* 2 (August) 8035:417–18.

Marchesini, G., R. Marzocchi, F. Agostini, and E. Bugianesi. 2005. Nonalcoholic fatty liver disease and the metabolic syndrome. *Curr Opin Lipidol* 16 (August) 4:421–27.

Maric, R. 2000. Meat intake, heterocyclic amines, and colon cancer *Am J Gastroenterol* 95 (December) 12:3683–84.

Marshall, K. 2000. Population-based fecal occult blood screening for colon cancer: Will the benefits outweigh the harm? *CMAJ* 163 (September) 5:545–46.

Mattson, M. P., and F. Haberman. 2003. Folate and homocysteine metabolism: therapeutic targets in cardiovascular and neurodegenerative disorders. *Curr Med Chem* 10(19): 1923–29.

Maudgal, D. P. 1991. A practical guide to the nonsurgical treatment of gallstones. *Drugs* 41 (February) 2:185–92.

Maxwell, S. R, and D. J. Webb. 2005. COX-2 selective inhibitors: iImportant lessons learned. *Lancet* 365 (February) 9458:449–51.

McArthur, K. E. 1988. Soy protein meals stimulate less gastric acid secretion and gastrin release than beef meals. *Gastroenterology* 95(4): 920–26.

Meningaud, J. P., F. Bado, E. Favre, J. C. Bertrand, and F. Guilbert. 1999. *Rev Stomatol Chir Maxillofac* 100(5): 240–44.

Meshikhes, A. W. 2002. Asymptomatic gallstones in the laparoscopic era. *J R Coll Surg Edinb* 47 (December) 6:742–48.

Midgley, R. 1999. Colorectal cancer. *Lancet* 353 (January) 9150:391–99.

Millward, C., M. Ferriter, S. Calver, and G. Connell-Jones. 2004. Gluten- and casein-free diets for autistic spectrum disorder. *Cochrane Database Syst Rev* 2:CD003498.

Milton, K. 1999. A hypothesis to explain the role of meat-eating in human evolution. *Evol Anthropol* 8:11–21.

———. 2000a. Back to basics: Why foods of wild primates have relevance for modern human health. *Nutrition* 16 (July–August) 7–8:480–83.

———. 2000b. Hunter-gatherer diets: A different perspective. *Am J Clin Nutr* 71 (Mar) 3:665–67.

Misciagna, G. 2000. Diet and duodenal ulcer. *Dig Liver Dis* 32 (August– September) 6:468–72.

Moayyedi, P., S. Soo, J. Deeks, B. Delaney, A. Harris, M. Innes, R. Oakes, S. Wilson, A. Roalfe, C. Bennett, and D. Forman. 2005. Eradication of *Helicobacter pylori* for non-ulcer dyspepsia. *Cochrane Database Syst Rev* (January) 1:CD002096.

Montrose, D. C, and M. H. Floch. 2005. Probiotics used in human studies. *J Clin Gastroenterol* 39 (July) 6:469–84.

Moran, S. 1997. Effects of fiber administration in the prevention of gallstones in obese patients on a reducing diet: A clinical trial. *Rev Gastroenterol Mex* 62 (October–December) 4:266–72.

Morson, B. 1976. Genesis of colonrectal cancer. *Clin Gastroenterol* 5:505.

Murphy, D. 1988. Chocolate and heartburn: evidence of increased esophageal acid exposure after chocolate ingestion. *Am J Gastroenterol* 83(6): 633–36.

Naaeder, S. B. 1998. Acute appendicitis and dietary fibre intake. *West Afr J Med* 17 (October–December) 4:264–67.

Nagase, M., H. Tanimura, M. Setoyama, and Y. Hikasa. 1978. Present features of gallstones in Japan: A collective review of 2,144 cases. *Am J Surg* 135 (June) 6:788–90.

Nair, P., and J. F. Mayberry. 1994. Vegetarianism, dietary fibre and gastro-intestinal disease. *Dig Dis* 12 (May–June) 3:177–85.

Nanda, R. 1989. Food intolerance and the irritable bowel syndrome. *Gut* 30 (August) 8:1099–104.

Nasset, E. 1961. Movements of the small intestine. P. Bard. *Medical Physiology* 11 ed., 440. St. Louis: C. V. Mosby.

National Institute for Health Care Management. 2002. Prescription drug expenditures in the year 2001: Another year of escalating costs. (revised May 6, 2002) http://www.nihcm.org/spending2001.pdf.

Nebel, O. 1976. Symptomatic gastroesophageal reflux: Incidence and precipitating factors. *Am J Dig Dis* 21:953–56.

Nestle, M. 1999. Animal v. plant foods in human diets and health: Is the historical record unequivocal? *Proc Nutr Soc* 58 (May) 2:211–18.

Niec, A. M. 1998. Are adverse food reactions linked to irritable bowel syndrome? *Am J Gastroenterol* 93 (November) 11:2184–90.

Niedzielin, K. 2001. A controlled, double-blind, randomized study on the efficacy of *Lactobacillus plantarum* 299V in patients with irritable bowel syndrome. *Eur J Gastroenterol Hepatol* 13 (October) 10:1143–47.

Njelekela, M., T. Sato, Y. Nara, T. Miki, S. Kuga, T. Noguchi, T. Kanda, M. Yamori, J. Ntogwisangu, Z. Masesa, Y. Mashalla, J. Mtabaji, and Y. Yamori. 2003. Nutritional variation and cardiovascular risk factors in Tanzania: Rural-urban difference. *S Afr Med J* 93 (April) 4:295–99.

Nobaek, S. 2000. Alteration of intestinal microflora is associated with reduction in abdominal bloating and pain in patients with irritable bowel syndrome. *Am J Gastroenterol* 95 (May) 5:1231–38.

Norris, J. M, K. Barriga, E. J. Hoffenberg, I. Taki, D. Miao, J. E. Haas, L. M. Emery, R. J. Sokol, H. A. Erlich, G. S. Eisenbarth, and M. Rewers. 2005. Risk of celiac disease autoimmunity and timing of gluten introduction in the diet of infants at increased risk of disease. *JAMA* 293 (May) 19:2343–51.

O'Donnell, L. J. 1999. Post-cholecystectomy diarrhoea: a running commentary. *Gut* 45 (December) 6:796–97.

O'Keefe, S. 1999. Rarity of colon cancer in Africans is associated with low animal product consumption, not fiber. *Am J Gastroenterol* 94 (May) 5:1373–80.

Oboh, H. 2000. Effect of soaking, cooking and germination on the oligosaccharide content of selected Nigerian legume seeds. *Plant Foods Hum Nutr* 55(2): 97–110.

Oeppen, R. S. 2003. Denis Parsons Burkitt (1911–1993). *Br J Oral Maxillofac Surg* 41 (August) 4:235.

Ogendo, S. W. 1991. A study of haemorrhoids as seen at the Kenyatta National Hospital with special reference to asymptomatic haemorrhoids. *East Afr Med J* 68 (May) 5:340–47.

Painter, N. 1975. Diverticular disease of the colon, a 20th century problem. *Clin Gastroenterol* 4 (January) 1:3–21.

Palmer, R. H. 2003. Alosetron for irritable bowel syndrome: Risks of using alosetron are still unknown. *BMJ* 326 (January) 7379:51.

Parisi, G. C. 2002. High-fiber diet supplementation in patients with irritable bowel syndrome (IBS): A multicenter, randomized, open trial comparison between wheat bran diet and partially hydrolyzed guar gum (PHGG). *Dig Dis Sci* 47 (August) 8:1697–704.

Pehl, C. 1997. The effect of decaffeination of coffee on gastro-oesophageal reflux in patients with reflux disease. *Aliment Pharmacol Ther* 11(3): 483–86.

Peltonen, R., W. H. Lillg, O. Hanninen, and F. Ferola. 1992. An uncooked vegan diet shifts the profile of human fecal microflora: Computerized analysis of direct stool sample gas-liquid chromatography profiles of bacterial cellular fatty acids. *Appl Environ Microbiol* 58 (November) 11:3660–66.

Peltonen, R., M. Nenonen, T. Helve, O. Hanninen, P. Toivanen, and E. Eerola. 1997. Faecal microbial flora and disease activity in rheumatoid arthritis during a vegan diet. *Br J Rheumatol* 36 (January) 1:64–68.

Pennington, Jean A., Anna De Planter Bowes, and Helen Nichols Church. 1998. *Bowes & Church's food values of portions commonly used* 17th edition. Philadelphia and New York: Lippincott.

Pennisi, E. 1999. Did cooked tubers spur the evolution of big brains? *Science* 283 (March) 5410:2004–05.

Peters, H. P. 2001. Potential benefits and hazards of physical activity and exercise on the gastrointestinal tract. *Gut* 48 (March) 3:435–39.

Petroni, M.L. 2001. Ursodeoxycholic acid alone or with chenodeoxycholic acid for dissolution of cholesterol gallstones: a randomized multicentre trial: The British-Italian Gallstone Study group. *Aliment Pharmacol Ther* 15 (January) 1:123–28.

Picci, R., S. G. Perri, A. Dalla Torre, D. Pietrasanta, P. Castaldo, A. Nicita, M. Del Prete, M. Meli, and A. Moraldi A. 2005. Therapy of asymptomatic gallstones: indications and limits. *Chir Ital* 57 (January–February) 1:35–45.

Pickhardt, P. J. 2003. Computed tomographic virtual colonoscopy to screen for colorectal neoplasia in asymptomatic adults. *N Engl J Med* 349 (December) 23:2191–200.

Pignone, M. 2002. Screening for colorectal cancer in adults at average risk: A summary of the evidence for the U.S. Preventive Services Task Force. *Ann Intern Med* 137 (July) 2:132–41.

Pixley, F. 1985. Effect of vegetarianism on development of gall stones in women. *Br Med J (Clin Res Ed)* 291 (July) 6487:11–12.

Portincasa, P., A. Moschetta, K. J. van Erpecum, M. Vacca, M. Petruzzelli, G. Calamita, G. Meyer, and G. Palasciano. 2005. Modulation of cholesterol crystallization in bile: Implications for non-surgical treatment of cholesterol gallstone disease. *Curr Drug Targets Immune Endocr Metabol Disord* 5 (June) 2:177–84.

Potter, T. 1985. Activated charcoal: in vivo and in vitro studies of effect on gas formation. *Gastroenterology* 88 (March) 3:620–24.

Pounder, R. 2002. *Helicobacter pylori* and NSAIDs: The end of the debate? *Lancet* 358: 3–4.

Price, S. 1978. Food sensitivity in reflux esophagitis. *Am J Gastroenterol* 75:240–43.

Prosser, C. 1961. *Comparative Animal Physiology*, 2nd ed. Philadelphia: W. B. Saunders, 116.

Ransohoff, D. F. 1993. Treatment of gallstones. *Ann Intern Med* 119 (October) 7 Pt 1:606–19.

Ratcliff, P. A., and P. W. Johnson. 1999. The relationship between oral malodor, gingivitis, and periodontitis. *J Periodontol* 70 (5): 485–89.

Reddy, B. S., J. H. Weisburger, and E. L. Wynder. 1975. Effects of high risk and low risk diets for colon carcinogenesis on fecal microflora and steroids in man. *J Nutr* 105 (July) 7:878–84.

Reddy, B. S. 1998. Prevention of colon cancer by pre- and probiotics: Evidence from laboratory studies. *Br J Nutr* 80 (October) 4:S219–23.

———. 1999. Role of dietary fiber in colon cancer: an overview. *Am J Med* 106 (January) 1A:16S–19S.

Revicki, D. A. 1998. The impact of gastroesophageal reflux disease on health-related quality of life. *Am J Med* 104 (3): 252–58.

Rex, D. 1997. Colonoscopic miss rates of adenomas determined by back-to-back colonoscopies. *Gastroenterology* 112:24.

Riordan, A. M. 1993. Treatment of active Crohn's disease by exclusion diet: East Anglian multicentre controlled trial. *Lancet* 342 (November) 8880:1131–34.

Robins, G., and P. D. Howdle. 2005. Advances in celiac disease. *Curr Opin Gastroenterol* 21 (March) 2:152–61.

Rodriguez, S. 1998. Meal type affects heartburn severity. *Dig Dis Sci* 43 (3): 485–90.

Roediger, W. 1993. Sulphide impairment of substrate oxidation in rat colonocytes: A biochemical basis for ulcerative colitis? *Clin Sci (Lond)* 85 (November) 5:623–27.

Rubaltelli, F. F., R. Biadaioli, P. Pecile, and P. Nicoletti. 1998. Intestinal flora in breast- and bottle-fed infants. *J Perinat Med* 26 (3): 186–91.

Rush, E. C. 2002. Kiwifruit promotes laxation in the elderly. *Asia Pac J Clin Nutr* 11 (2): 164–68.

Sakamoto, N., S. Kono, K. Wakai, Y. Fukuda, M. Satomi, et al. 2005. Epidemiology Group of the Research Committee on Inflammatory Bowel Disease in Japan. Dietary risk factors for inflammatory bowel disease: A multicenter case-control study in Japan. *Inflamm Bowel Dis* 11 (February) 2:154–63.

Salminen, S. J, M. Gueimonde, and E. Isolauri. 2005. Probiotics that modify disease risk. *J Nutr* 135 (May) 5:1294–98.

Samuelsson, S. M. 1991. Risk factors for extensive ulcerative colitis and ulcerative proctitis: A population based case-control study. *Gut* 32 (December) 12:1526–30.

Sartor, R. B. 2005. Probiotic therapy of intestinal inflammation and infections. *Curr Opin Gastroenterol* 21 (January) 1:44–50.

Saunders, K. D. 1993. Lovastatin and gallstone dissolution: a preliminary study. *Surgery* 113 (January) 1:28–35.

Scheppach, W. 2001. Beneficial health effects of low-digestible carbohydrate consumption. *Br J Nutr* 85 Suppl 1:S23-30.

Schroeder, P. 1995. Dental erosion and acid reflux disease. *Ann Intrn Med* 122:809–15.

Segal, I. 2001. Persistent low prevalence of Western digestive diseases in Africa: Confounding aetiological factors. *Gut* 48 (May) 5:730–32.

———. 2002. Physiological small bowel malabsorption of carbohydrates protects against large bowel diseases in Africans. *J Gastroenterol Hepatol* 17 (March) 3:249–52.

Segasothy, M. 1999. Vegetarian diet: panacea for modern lifestyle? *Q J Med* 92:531–44.

Selby, J. 1992. A case-control study of screening sigmoidoscopy and mortality from colorectal cancer. *N Engl J Med* 326:653.

———. 1993. Screening sigmoidoscopy for colonrectal cancer. *Lancet* 341:728.

Serpick, A. A. 1976. Spontaneous regression of colon carcinoma. *Natl Cancer Inst Monogr*, November, 44:21.

Serraino, M. 1992. Flaxseed supplementation and early markers of colon carcinogenesis. *Cancer Lett* 63 (April) 2:159–65.

Shaffer, E. A. 2005. Epidemiology and risk factors for gallstone disease: Has the paradigm changed in the 21st century? *Curr Gastroenterol Rep* 7 (May) 2:132–40.

Shapiro, J. P. 2000. A pill turned bitter. How a quest for a blockbuster drug went fatally wrong. *US News World Rep* 129 (December) 23:54–56.

Shibata, M. A. 2003. Comparative effects of lovastatin on mammary and prostate oncogenesis in transgenic mouse models. *Carcinogenesis* 24 (Mar) 3:453–59.

Shike, M. 1999. Diet and lifestyle in the prevention of colorectal cancer: an overview. *Am J Med* 106 (January) 1A:11S–15S.

Simpson, J. 1995. Pathogenesis of colonic diverticula. *Br J Surg* 89 (May) 5:546–54.

Simpson, W. 1995. Gastroesophageal reflux disease and asthma: Diagnosis and management. *Arch Intrn Med* 155:798–803.

Singh, P. N. 1998. Dietary risk factors for colon cancer in a low-risk population. *Am J Epidemiol* 148 (October) 8:761–74.

Singh, D., and P. M. Bronstad. 2001. Female body odour is a potential cue to ovulation. *Proc Biol Sci* 22, 268 (1469): 797–801.

Sivan, G. 1997. *Helicobacter pylori*: In vitro susceptibility to garlic (Allium sativum) extract. *Nutr Cancer* 27:118–21.

Slattery, M. L. 2001. Trans-fatty acids and colon cancer. *Nutr Cancer* 39 (2): 170–75.

Smit, C. F. 2001. Effect of cigarette smoking on gastropharyngeal and gastroesophageal reflux. *Ann Otol Rhinol Laryngol* 110 (2): 190–93.

Smith M., L. G. Smith, and B. Levinson. 1982. The use of smell in differential diagnosis. *Lancet* 2(8313): 1452–53.

Sontag, S. J. 1999. Defining GERD. *Yale J Biol Med* 72 (March–June) 2–3:69–80.

Stacewicz-Sapuntzakis, M. 2001. Chemical composition and potential health effects of prunes: A functional food? *Crit Rev Food Sci Nutr* 41 (May) 4:251–86.

Story, J.A., and D. Kritchevsky. 1994. Denis Parsons Burkitt (1911-1993). *J Nutr* 124 (September) 9:1551–54.

Strasberg, S. 1998. The pathogenesis of cholesterol gallstones a review. *J Gastrointest Surg* 2 (March–April) 2:109–25.

Stryker, S. 1987. Natural history of untreated colonic polyps. *Gastroenterology* 93:1009.

Suadicani, P. 1999. Genetic and life-style determinants of peptic ulcer. A study of 3387 men aged 54 to 74 years. The Copenhagen Male Study. *Scand J Gastroenterol* 34 (January) 1:12–17.

Suarez F. 1998. Identification of gases responsible for the odour of human flatus and evaluation of a device purported to reduce this odour. *Gut* 43 (July) 1:100–04.

———. 1999. Failure of activated charcoal to reduce the release of gases produced by the colonic flora. *Am J Gastroenterol* 94 (January) 1:208–12.

Suarez F. L., J. K. Furne, J. Springfield, and M. D. Levitt. 2000. Morning breath odor: influence of treatments on sulfur gases. *J Dent Res* 79 (10): 1773–77.

Tabak, M., R. Armon, I. Potasman, and I. Neeman. 1996. In vitro inhibition of *Helicobacter pylori* by extracts of thyme. *J. Appl. Microbiol* 80:667–672.

Tasker, A., P. W. Dettmar, M. Panetti, J. A. Koufman, J. P. Birchall, and J. P. Pearson. 2002. Reflux of gastric juice and glue ear in children. *Lancet* 359 (9305): 493.

Taylor, R. 1990. Management of constipation: High fibre diets work. *BMJ* 300 (April) 6731:1063–64.

Tazuma, S. 1998. A combination therapy with simvastatin and ursodeoxycholic acid is more effective for cholesterol gallstone dissolution than is ursodeoxycholic acid monotherapy. *J Clin Gastroenterol* 26 (June) 4:287–91.

Teyssen, S. 1999. Maleic acid and succinic acid in fermented alcoholic beverages are the stimulants of gastric acid secretion. *J Clin Invest* 103 (March) 5:707–13.

Thompson, W. G. 2003. Diverticula, seeds and nuts. *Digestive Health Mattersi*, Summer.

Thyagarajan, S. P. 1988. Effect of Phyllanthus amarus on chronic carriers of hepatitis B virus. *Lancet* 2 (October) 8614:764–66.

Toivanen, P., and E. Eerola. 2002. A vegan diet changes the intestinal flora. *Rheumatology* (Oxford). 41 (August) 8:950–51.

Tomlin, L. 1991. Investigation of normal flatus production in healthy volunteers. *Gut* 32 (June) 6:665–69.

Tragnone, A. 1995. Dietary habits as risk factors for inflammatory bowel disease. *Eur J Gastroenterol Hepatol* 7 (January) 1:47–51.

Truelove, S. 1961. Ulcerative colitis provoked by milk. *Br Med J* 1:154.

Tsai, C. J., M. F. Leitzmann, W. C. Willett, and E. L. Giovannucci. 2004. Long-term intake of dietary fiber and decreased risk of cholecystectomy in women. *Am J Gastroenterol* 99 (July) 7:1364–70.

Tseng, M. 1999. Dietary intake and gallbladder disease: A review. *Public Health Nutr* 2 (June) 2:161–72.

Tyagi, K. 1974. Gastric mucosal morphology in tropics and influence of spices, tea, and smoking. *Nutr Metab* 17:129–35.

Ueno, T. 1997. Therapeutic effects of restricted diet and exercise in obese patients with fatty liver. *J Hepatol* 27 (July) 1:103–07.

Ung, K. A, R. Gillberg, A. Kilander, and H. Abrahamsson. 2000. Role of bile acids and bile acid binding agents in patients with collagenous colitis. *Gut* 46 (February) 2:170–05.

Uribe, M. 1982. Treatment of chronic portal: Systemic encephalopathy with vegetable and animal protein diets. A controlled crossover study. *Dig Dis Sci* 27 (December) 12:1109–16.

Vajro, P. 1994. Persistent hyperaminotransferasemia resolving after weight reduction in obese children. *J Pediatr* 125 (August) 2:239–41.

Van Deventer, G. 1992. Lower esophageal sphincter pressure, acid secretion, and blood gastrin after coffee consumption. *Dig Dis Sci* 37 (4): 558–69.

Viljamaa, M., K. Kaukinen, H. Huhtala, S. Kyronpalo, M. Rasmussen, and P. Collin. 2005. Coeliac disease, autoimmune diseases and gluten exposure. *Scand J Gastroenterol* 40 (April) 4:437–43.

Walker, A. 1973. Appendicitis, fibre intake and bowel behaviour in ethnic groups in South Africa. *Postgrad Med J* 49 (April) 570:243–49.

———. 1979. Epidemiology of noninfective intestinal diseases in various ethnic groups in South Africa. *Isr J Med Sci* 15 (April) 4:309–13.

Weinberg, D. 1996. The diagnosis and management of gastroesophageal reflux disease. *Med Clin North Am* 80 (2): 411–29.

Weisburger, J. H. 2000. Eat to live, not live to eat. *Nutrition* 16 (9): 767–73.

Wendl, B. 1994. Effect of decaffeination of coffee or tea on gastro-oesophageal reflux. *Aliment Pharmacol Ther* 8 (3): 283–87.

Westman, E.C. 2002. Effect of 6-month adherence to a very low carbohydrate diet program. *Am J Med* 113 (July) 1:30–36.

Ananda Marga Publications. 1977. *What's Wrong with Eating Meat?* New Delhi: Ananda Marga Publications.

Wheeler, J. G, S. J. Shema, M. L. Bogle, M. A. Shirrell, A. W. Burks, A. Pittler, and R. M. Helm. 1997. Immune and clinical impact of Lactobacillus acidophilus on asthma. *Ann Allergy Asthma Immunol* 79 (September) 3:229–33.

Winawer, S. J. 1993. Randomized comparison of surveillance intervals after colonoscopic removal of newly diagnosed adenomatous polyps. The National Polyp Study Workgroup. *N Engl J Med* 328 (April) 13:901–06.

———. 1999. Natural history of colorectal cancer. *Am J Med* 106 (January) 1A:3S–6S.

———. 2000. A comparison of colonoscopy and double-contrast barium enema for surveillance after polypectomy. National Polyp Study Work Group. *N Engl J Med* 342 (June) 24:1766–72.

Wisten, A., and T. Messner. 2005. Fruit and fibre (Pajala porridge) in the prevention of constipation. *Scand J Caring Sci* 19 (March) 1:71–76.

Wood, B. 1999. Human evolution: We are what we ate. *Nature* 400:219–20.

Workman, E. M. 1984. Diet in the management of Crohn's disease. *Hum Nutr Appl Nutr* 38 (December) 6:469–73.

Wright, R. 1965. A controlled therapeutic trial of various diets in ulcerative colitis. *Br Med J* 22:138–41.

———. 1965. Circulating antibodies to dietary proteins in ulcerative colitis. *Br Med J* 2:142–44.

Yaegaki, K., and J. M. Coil. 2000. Examination, classification, and treatment of halitosis; clinical perspectives. *J Can Dent Assoc* 66:257–61.

Yamashiki, M. 1997. Effects of the Japanese herbal medicine "Sho-saiko-to" (TJ-9) on in vitro interleukin-10 production by peripheral blood mononuclear cells of patients with chronic hepatitis C. *Hepatology* 25 (June) 6:1390–97.

Yang, H. 1992. Risk factors for gallstone formation during rapid loss of weight. *Dig Dis Sci* 37 (June) 6:912–18.

Young-Fadok, T. Epidemiology and pathophysiology of colonic diverticular disease. http://www.uptodate.com/patient_info/topicpages/topics/6088F9.asp

Zar, S. 2001. Food hypersensitivity and irritable bowel syndrome. *Aliment Pharmacol Ther* 15 (April) 4:439–49.

Zubler, J., G. Markowski, S. Yale, R. Graham, and T. C. Rosenthal. 1998. Natural history of asymptomatic gallstones in family practice office practices. *Arch Fam Med* 7 (May–June) 3:230–33.

Index

acarbose, 133
acid reflux. *See* gastroe-
    sophageal reflux
    disease
acidophilus, 123. *See also*
    Lactobacilli bacteria
Actigall, 57–58
adaptive response, 15
aflatoxins, 66
African diet, 81–84, 88,
    109
alcoholic beverages,
    28–29, 43, 61, 62
alosetron, 95
alpha-amylase, 137–38
amino acids, 101
anaerobic bacteria, 19
anal fissures, 74
antacids, 24, 33, 41
antiulcerants, 24
appendicitis, 83–84
appendix, 83, 84
arthritis, 44
aspirin, 40, 42, 43
asthma, 31–32
autoimmune diseases, 97,
    98

bacteria. *See* bowel bacte-
    ria; *Helicobacter
    pylori*

bad breath, 11, 22
    diet and, 14–15
    and health, 21
    sulfur compounds and,
        17–21
    teethbrushing and,
        18–20
    types of, 16–18
baking without oil, 154
barium enema, 111, 113
Beano, 131
beans, 130, 144
    "degassing," 130, 131
beer, 29, 43
Bifidobacterium, 120, 122
bile, 50–52, 56, 57, 102,
    110
blood sugar, elevated, 122
body odor, 12–13, 22
    diet and, 13–15
bowel bacteria, beneficial,
    117–19, 124–25. *See
    also* Lactobacilli
    bacteria
    beginnings of good
        bacteria, 119–20
    benefits of, 117–19,
        124
    diet and, 120–21
    probiotic supplements
        and, 96, 121–24

bowel movements, 69–70,
    80
    frequency, 71
    gone bad, 71–72
    normal, 70–71
bowel sickness. *See also*
    specific disorders
    fiber and, 81–83,
        91–92
    treatment of damaged
        tissues, 91
bran, 78, 110, 111
bread. *See also* wheat
    sourdough, 98
breast-feeding, 120, 124
breath odor. *See* bad
    breath
broccoli, 46
Burkitt, Denis, 81–84, 109

cabbage juice, 46
cancer. *See also* colon
    cancer
    diet and, 109–10
candida, 122
capsaicin, 40
celiac disease, 96–98
    diet as only treatment
        for, 99–100
    foods acceptable for,
        99

health problems more
common with, 97, 98
offending foods for, 97,
98
charcoal, activated, 131
chenodeoxycholic acid
(CDCA), 57
chocolate, 29
choking, 137
cholecystectomy, 55–57
cholesterol:
dietary, 138–39
elevated blood, 122
cholesterol gallstones,
51–53, 57–58, 139
cigarette smoking, 28–29
cirrhosis, 61, 63
citrus fruits, 29
coffee, 28
colitis, 21, 93–94, 106. See
also ulcerative colitis
dietary treatment, 96,
101–06
mild/chronic/spastic,
96 (see also irritable
bowel syndrome)
severe, 100–02
colon, spastic, 94
colon cancer, 107–09, 122
causes and progression
of, 108–11
diet and, 109–10
fiber and, 110–11
screening for, 111–14
treatment of, 114
colon disease. See also
polyps
progression, 108, 114
treatment, 114
colon health, fiber and,
110–11
colonoscopy:
optical, 112
virtual, 113
constipation, 71–72, 80

causes:
dairy products,
72–73, 75
uncommon, 74–75
consequences of, 26–27
fiber and, 75–77
irritable bowel syn-
drome and, 94
treatment, 77–80, 122
cooking tools, 152
cookware, 152
Crohn's disease (CD),
100–102, 122
cruciferous vegetables, 46
cyclooxygenase (COX), 43
cyclooxygenase-2 (COX-2)
inhibitors, 43–44
cysteine, 18

dairy, 41, 147. See also milk
and constipation,
72–73, 75
and flatulence, 128
as a source of probiotics,
123
and ulcers, 40–41
dental erosions, 31
dental health, 122. See
also oral hygiene
dermatitis, atopic, 122
diabetes, 122
diaphragm, 89
diarrhea, 93–94, 122. See
also colitis; irritable
bowel syndrome
diet(s), 141. See also nutrition; specific topics
cross-cultural compari-
son of, 7–8, 81–84,
88, 109
high-fat, 28
importance, 3
societies with plant-
based, high-
carbohydrate, 7–8

digestive system, 9–10,
137–38
digital rectal examination
(DRE), 112
dihydrogen sulfide (H_2S),
17
diverticula, 85–86
diverticular disease,
84–86, 122
drug companies, 95
dyspepsia. See heartburn

eczema, 122
eggs, 41
intolerance to, 96
elemental diets, 101
elimination diet, 103–05
enemas, rectal, 79
esophageal sphincter. See
lower esophageal
sphincter

fast food, 32
fat intake, 53, 83, 101,
102, 147
fatty infiltration of the
liver, 63–64
fiber, 27, 75–76, 80, 128
and bowel health, 27,
75–77, 80–92, 96,
110–11
and gallstones, 52
soluble and insoluble,
110
fiber supplements, 78
flatulence, 127–34
causes, 133
cooking methods to
reduce, 131
gassy foods, 128, 130
sex differences in,
129
flaxseeds, 78
flora. See bowel bacteria;
Lactobacilli bacteria

About the Author

John A. McDougall, MD, has been studying, writing, and "speaking out" about the effects of nutrition on disease for over 30 years. One of his fundamental beliefs is that people are supposed to look, function, and feel great, and enjoy optimal health for a lifetime—if that's not the case, they need to change their lifestyle. Dr. McDougall's role is to educate people so they can improve their lives.

He is the founder and medical director of the nationally renowned residential 10-day McDougall Program, located at a luxury resort in Santa Rosa, California. Thousands of his patients [ov]er the last three decades of his medical practice have been able [to el]iminate all unnecessary medications, while regaining their health.

[A]s with many leaders, Dr. McDougall often finds it necessary [to ch]allenge accepted wisdom. He was one of the first traditional [physi]cians to claim that following a pure vegetarian diet can [cure] unfavorable medical conditions such as heart disease, diabetes, hypertension, arthritis, and obesity. Published [...]research and clinical results have solidly confirmed his

[A gra]duate of Michigan State University's College of Human [Medicine, h]e performed his internship at Queen's Medical Center in [Honolulu, H]awaii, and his medical residency at the University of [Hawaii. He is] board certified as a specialist in Internal Medicine by [American] Board of Internal Medicine and is certified by the [...]d of Medical Examiners.

food, a new way of thinking about, 7–10
food allergies, 75. *See also* elimination diet
food ingredients, 147
food intolerances, 96, 102. *See also* celiac disease
food pantry. *See* pantry
freezer, well-stocked, 151
fruit, 78, 145, 151
fruit juice vs. whole fruit, 29

gallbladder, 50, 59
　diet and, 53
　function and purpose, 50, 56
gallbladder attacks, 49–52
gallbladder disease, 49, 59
gallstones, 49, 50, 59, 139
　dissolving, 57–58
　prescription for, 52–55
　strategies for treatment and management of, 55
　disadvantages of surgery, 56–57
　"expectant management," 55, 56, 58
　immediate surgery, 55–56
　weight loss and, 53–54
gastritis, 44
gastroesophageal endoscopy, 24
gastroesophageal reflux disease (GERD), 24–26, 35. *See also* lower esophageal sphincter (LES) dysfunction
　acid damage from the teeth to the lungs, 30–32

diet, constipation, and, 26–27, 32, 34, 35
　medications for treatment of, 32–34
gingivitis, 20. *See also* periodontal disease
gluten, 96–99
grains and grain products, 144
guar gum, partially hydrolyzed, 78

H₂ receptor antagonists, 33–34
halitosis. *See also* bad breath
　and health, 21
　pathologic, 16–17
　physiologic, 16–18
heart attacks, 82–83
heartburn, 23. *See also* gastroesophageal reflux disease; lower esophageal sphincter (LES) dysfunction causes, 32
Helicobacter pylori (H. pylori), 44–46, 122
hemorrhoids, 74, 86–88, 114–15
　treatment, 87
hepatitis. *See also* steatohepatitis
　infectious, 64–65, 68
　drug therapies for, 66
　herbs for, 65–66
hepatitis C, 64–65
hernia, 90
　hiatus (hiatal), 26–27, 89–90

immobility and constipation, 74
immunity, 122
indigestion. *See* heartburn

infants, 119–20, 122, 124
inflammatory bowel disease (IBD), 100, 106
　dietary causes, 100–101, 106
interferon, 66
intestines, 8, 9, 102, 138. *See also* large intestine
irritable bowel syndrome (IBS), 72, 94, 106, 122. *See also* celiac disease; colitis
　drug therapy for, 95
　fiber and, 96
　predominant diarrhea vs. constipation-type, 96
　probiotics and, 132
　symptoms, 94

Jianpi Wenshen recipe, 65–66
joint pain, 44

kitchen tools, 152

lactitol, 123
Lactobacilli bacteria, 96, 98, 122, 123, 132. *See also* bowel bacteria
lactose, 128
lactose intolerance, 128, 130
lactulose, 123, 133
laparoscopic cholecystectomy, 55–57
large intestine, 83–85, 102. *See also* intestines
　as microbial factory, 118–19
laxatives, 78

and constipation, 74, 77

"lazy bowel," 77

limbic system, 13, 14

liver, 68
cholesterol and, 138–39
as detoxifier, 61–64
diet and, 61, 138–39

liver disease, 61, 62, 68
fatty, 63–64

liver enzymes, elevated, 64, 66

liver-toxic chemicals, 66

liver-toxic drugs, 67

Lotronex, 95

lower esophageal sphincter (LES), 25–26, 90

lower esophageal sphincter (LES) dysfunction, 25, 26, 35. *See also* gastroesophageal reflux disease
causes of long-term, 26–27
causes of short-term, 26–29
medications that can cause, 33

McDougall, Mary, 103, 144, 155

McDougall Diet. *See also* *specific topics*
foods not allowed, 145–46
foods to enjoy, 144–46

McDougall Quick and Easy Cookbook, 153

McDougall Web site, v, 153

methionine, 18

methyl mercaptan (CH3SH), 17, 21

microbial putrefaction, 17

microflora. See bowel bacteria; Lactobacilli bacteria

milk. *See also* dairy
allergy to protein in cow's, 75
intolerance to, 96
and ulcers, 40–41

milk thistle, 66

morning breath, 19, 20.
See also bad breath

mouthwash, 19, 20

nitrosamines, 66

nonsteroidal anti-inflammatory drugs (NSAIDs). *See also* aspirin
toxic damage from, 42–45

nutrition, 141. *See also* diet(s); *specific topics*
body's need for plant nutrients, 139–40
what anatomy says about, 137
what evolution says about, 136
what our digestive system says about, 137–38

obesity, 64

occult blood test, 112

olfactory lobes, 13, 14

oligosaccharides, 121, 123. *See also* prebiotics

onions, 29

oral hygiene, 16, 18–22.
See also bad breath

osmotic agents, 79

packaged foods, 150

pantry:
fresh foods for, 150
well-stocked, 148–50

pantry shelf staples, 148–49

partially hydrolyzed guar gum (PHGG), 78

pepper, 39, 40

periodontal disease, 20, 21

Phyllanthus amarus, 65

plant nutrients. *See also* nutrition; *specific topics*
body's need for, 139–40
human instinct for, 139

polyps, 108
and colon cancer, 108
diet and, 109–11
screening for, 111–14

potatoes, mashed, 143–44

prebiotics, 121, 122

premenstrual syndrome (PMS), 122

probiotics, 96, 123. *See also* bowel bacteria
conditions aided by specific, 122
and flatulence, 132–33
when to take, 124

prostaglandins, 43

protein (intake), 63, 130, 135
animal vs. plant, 42, 63

proton pump inhibitors, 33, 34

ptyalin, 137–38

raffinose, 130, 131

recipes, where to find, 153

reflux. *See* gastroesophageal reflux disease

refrigerator, well-stocked, 150, 151

reproductive anatomy and vegetarian diet, 140

rheumatoid arthritis, 122

ribavirin, 66

sautéing without oil, 154–55

Schneider, George, 19

seasonings, 151, 153. *See also* spicy foods

seminal vesicles, 140

sexual desire, smell and, 13

Sho-saiko-to, 66

shopping habits, healthful, 147–55

sigmoid/barium enema, 111, 113

sigmoidoscopy exam, 112

Sippy Diet, 41

small intestine, 102. *See also* intestines

smells. *See also* body odor; flatulence
significance of, 12–13

snack foods, 152

sourdough bread, 98

spastic colon, 94. *See also* colitis; irritable bowel syndrome

spicy foods. *See also* seasonings
and ulcers, 39–40

sprouting beans, 131

stachyose, 130, 131

starches, 143–44. *See also* *specific topics*

steatohepatitis, nonalcoholic, 63–64

stimulants, 78

stomach, 38

stomach acid, 23–25, 28, 30, 38–39, 47. *See also* gastroesophageal reflux disease; lower esophageal sphincter (LES) dysfunction
alcohol and, 42–43
animal protein and, 42, 138
dairy products and, 41

stool bulking agents, 78

stools:
color, 71
consistency, 70, 71

sulfur compounds, gaseous, 17–21, 101, 110, 128

suppositories, rectal, 79

synbiotics, 123

teethbrushing and bad breath, 18–20

tongue, 19
cleaning the, 20

travel and constipation, 75

ulcerative colitis (UC), 100–02, 122

ulcers, 37–39, 46,
alcohol and, 4

animal foods and, 40–42

antibiotics for, 45–46

H. pylori bacteria and, 44–46, 122

NSAIDs and, 42–45

spicy foods and, 39–40

stress and, 39

ursodeoxycholic acid (UDCA), 57

uterus, prolapsed, 90, 91

vagotomy, 39

varicose veins, 88–89

vegetables, 144, 153
browning, without 153
cooking, 29
fresh, 150

vegetarian diet 139–41
specif
anatom
evolu
vitami
vitar

About the Artist

Howard C. Bartner retired in 2000 as Chief of Medical Illustration, Medical Art and Photography Branch, at the National Institutes of Health after 42 years of service. He received the NIH Director's Award for his outstanding contribution of medical illustrations for research scientists at the NIH. He is also the recipient of the Ranice W. Crosby Distinguished Achievement Medal from the Johns Hopkins University School of Medicine. As a graduate of the medical and biological program of the Johns Hopkins School of Medicine, he holds a teaching appointment as Associate Professor.

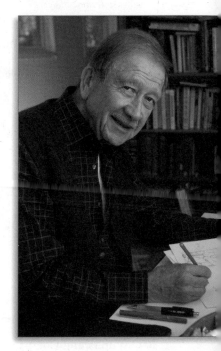

I met Howard in the summer of 2002 on a McDougall Adventure cruise to Alaska. My simple scrawls during daily lectures motivated Howard to help me communicate my medical messages more clearly. In return I had the opportunity to help him solve some serious health problems. We have been friends ever since that meeting and have worked together over the past four years to bring Larry and Louise to our readers. Howard's enjoyment of life and crisp sense of humor shine through these characters.

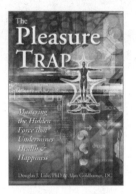
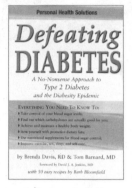
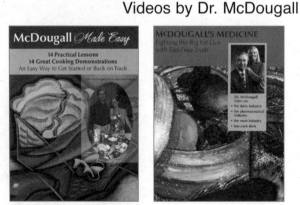
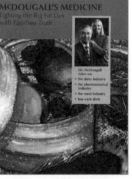
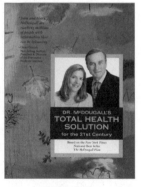